The Dancer Prepares

JAMES PENROD, M.F.A., has performed as a dancer and actor and has choreographed nationally and internationally in venues that include concert, theater, opera, and television. His work has been performed at renowned festivals in Edinburgh (Scotland), The Hague and Rotterdam (Holland), and Spoleto (Italy); by opera companies such as Opera Pacific and San Francisco; and for BBC II and NBC television. He has written two books and contributed numerous articles to national journals. As an administrator, he was a founding faculty member of the prestigious dance department at the University of California, Irvine, and served as the department chair for many years. He has also been associate dean for the Claire Trevor School of the Arts.

JANICE GUDDE PLASTINO, PH.D., is professor of dance at the University of California, Irvine, and teaches injury prevention, dance conditioning, kinesiology, tap, modern dance, and choreography. She has published on the subjects of dance medicine/science and dance education. She is on the editorial board for the *Journal of Dance Medicine and Science* and a member of the board of directors for Performing Arts Medicine Association and Music Intelligence Neural Development Institute (M.I.N.D.). She has performed and choreographed nationally and internationally. She was codirector of Penrod Plastino Movement Theatre for fifteen years. She established the first dance science emphasis in education at UCI in 1987 in cooperation with other health professionals. She was the 1991 NDA Dance Scholar and the 2001 Dance Teacher of the year.

Penrod and Plastino toured and danced as partners nationally and internationally with the dance company they formed in 1971, the Penrod Plastino Movement Theatre.

Higher Education

THE DANCER PREPARES, FIFTH EDITION

Published by McGraw-Hill, a business unit of The McGraw-Hill Companies, Inc., 1221 Avenue of the Americas, New York, NY, 10020. Copyright © 2005 by The McGraw-Hill Companies, Inc. All rights reserved. No part of this publication may be reproduced or distributed in any form or by any means, or stored in a database or retrieval system, without the prior written consent of The McGraw-Hill Companies, Inc., including, but not limited to, in any network or other electronic storage or transmission, or broadcast for distance learning.

1 2 3 4 5 6 7 8 9 0 DOC/DOC 0 9 8 7 6 5 4

ISBN 0-07-255726-5

www.mhhe.com

Library of Congress Cataloging-in-Publication Data

Penrod, James.
    The dancer prepares ; modern dance for beginners / James Penrod, Janice Gudde Plastino. — 5th ed.
        p. cm.
    Includes index.
    ISBN 0-07-255726-5 (softcover)
        1. Modern dance.   I. Plastino, Janice Gudde.   II. Title.

GV1783.P44 2004
792.8 — dc22

                                                                    2004049885

Publisher, William R. Glass; executive editor, Nicholas R. Barrett; director of development, Kathleen Engelberg; production editor, Jennifer Chambliss; developmental editor, Kathleen Naylor; production supervisor, Tandra Jorgensen; cover designer, Violeta Díaz; art editor, Katherine McNab; photo researcher, Natalia Peschiera. The text was set in 10/13 Minion by ColorType, San Diego, and printed on acid-free 45# New Era Matte by R. R. Donnelley in Crawfordsville, IN.

Cover Photo © 1994 Lois Greenfield. Illustrations based on drawings by Robert Carr. Additional photo credits appear at the back of the book on page 134, which constitutes an extension of the copyright page.

The Dancer Prepar

MODERN DANCE FOR BEGINN

Fifth Edition

James Penrod
Janice Gudde Plastino
University of California, Irvine

Boston   Burr Ridge, IL   Dubuque, IA   Madison, WI
San Francisco   St. Louis   Bangkok   Bogotá   Caracas
Lisbon   London   Madrid   Mexico City   Milan   Montre
Santiago   Seoul   Singapore   Sydney   Taipei

Contents

Preface

Dance is Movement that Lights the Soul.

— DONALD MCKAYLE

My Art is just an effort to express the truth of my Being in gesture and movement.

— ISADORA DUNCAN

In the dance . . . movement is its essence, its keynote and its language.

— DORIS HUMPHREY

Movement never lies. Everything that a dancer does on the stage tells the audience what he is.

— MARTHA GRAHAM

Dance includes every way men of all races, in every period of the world's history, have moved rhythmically to express themselves . . . understanding of the basic meanings of movement enable the creative dancer to take a significant, meaningful human gesture, and abstract and develop that into a dance . . . because all human movement is rooted in the universal human experience, and no one can arbitrarily change the basic meanings of movement.

— TED SHAWN

This book is written for you who are taking your first course in modern dance to introduce you to the content of the course and explain your role as a student. The authors assume you have little or no background in the art or technique of the dance.

No one can be taught how to be an artist, but you can be taught the craft of an art form. We hope to help you discover a new appreciation of the arts in general and to inspire in you a desire for self-discovery, self-discipline, and eventually self-expression in the art form of dance. This book introduces you to rudiments of the dancer's craft, such as basic techniques, dance clothes, and the care of your body. It also discusses choreographic fundamentals and evaluation procedures. We hope these objective principles will help you form a subjective ideal that will inspire you to commit yourself more fully to the dance world.

Why you have decided to study modern dance is of little consequence. The important thing is that you have enrolled in a course to learn the most exciting of the movement forms. You have chosen a course that is physically rigorous and at times satisfactorily exhausting; mentally stimulating and exasperating when the right solution to a challenge must be found; and creatively exciting and frustrating when the right creative moments have to be nudged, coaxed, and nurtured to come to a significant new life. It is probably one of the most self-satisfying courses that you will take. We do not assume that you will become a professional dancer, although we have directed the ideas in this book toward that goal. We do, however, hope you will experience the joy of movement well-executed, the exhilaration of creative endeavor, and the appreciation of dance—the most fleeting of the art forms.

This book is concerned primarily with the analysis of modern-dance techniques, combinations, and vocabulary. Although it is written for the beginning student, the book contains information that will be of value to the intermediate student as well.

This fifth edition has been updated and expanded with practical, theoretical, and historical information that will increase the usefulness of the book. In addition, key words in the text have been highlighted and included in a glossary at the end of the book for easy access to basic ideas introduced in the text. Selected websites have been added at the end of the book for those wanting further information on a particular dance subject. Selected references at the end of the book have been expanded. New photographs and artwork have been added.

Following is a description of some of the additions to this new edition.

Chapter One, Introduction

Dance careers are given greater coverage in this edition. A brief discussion of male and female contributions to modern dance is included, along with an expansion on the definition of modern dance with specific examples. We make suggestions on choosing dance performances to attend and how to evaluate and write about the performance.

Chapter Two, Preparation

Current ideas about dance clothing have been updated, and an overview of the history of dance costume is covered. Suggestions are also added for the warm-up and cool-down periods of a dance class, as well as the role of improvisation in class. There is now expanded coverage on the role of music in the classroom. Additional ideas on the purpose of the classroom critique from the teacher are presented, along with a significant number of ideas on critical self-assessment.

Chapter Three, Technique Analysis

Many boldface key terms and some expansion on key ideas, along with new floor schema for group work, have been added to this chapter.

Chapter Four, Anatomy, Injuries, and Diet

This chapter now includes updated information on dance as it relates to dance science, including warm-up and cool-down and injury prevention.

Chapter Five, History

We have added a highly informative new graph, which selectively shows a family tree of historical connections from early modern dance to contemporary. The chapter includes updated history and trends in the twenty-first century, with the inclusion of new artists and historical dates of leading dance figures.

Chapter Six, Improvisation

We discuss ideas on structured and nonstructured improvisation and give some background on Contact Improvisation.

Chapter Seven, Choreographic Approaches

Ideas related to theatrical elements of costumes, props, scenery, lighting, and sound are discussed. This chapter also provides suggestions on how to evaluate your own choreographic process and self-assessment.

Chapter Eight, Evaluation and Criticism

This chapter provides new insights and methods to evaluate and critically review dance — both your own and that of others.

Appendixes, Glossary, References

New pedagogical additions to the text include Appendix I on self-assessment, Appendix II with selected websites, boldface key terms in each chapter, a glossary of key terms, and updates on references.

We do not intend to preach a philosophy or theory of some ephemeral art form that can be mastered by reading statements about how to dance. We do intend to deal with concrete, specific, practical matters relating to the mastery of the creative and technical aspects of dance.

We would like to acknowledge the following individuals and institutions for their assistance: Norman Beede, Melanie A. Buchanan, Jennifer Fisher, William Landis, Loretta Livingston, Rita Marks, Susan McGreevy-Nichols and Helene Scheff, Donald McKayle, James Pleumer, Nancy Ruyter, and Lorelai Tanji. We would like to thank the reviewers: Elizabeth A. Smigel, University of Maryland; Jeanne Fornarola, University of Buffalo; Linda Roberts Alexanderson, Montclair State University; and Jodi Youmans-Jones, Casper College; as well as the many teachers who have suggested ideas for the book. We would like to extend appreciation to the University of California Dance Department and Special Collections and Archives at UC Irvine.

To
Robert Carr
Richard J. Plastino
Colleen Collins Smith

Chapter 1

Introduction

Love the art in yourself, rather than yourself in art.

STANISLAVSKY

Bebe Miller Company, The Hendrix Project. *Photo © 1995 Lois Greenfield.*

DEFINING MODERN DANCE

Modern dance is a performing dance art developed in the twentieth century by pioneers such as Isadora Duncan and Ruth St. Denis with an emphasis on the individual point of view in all aspects — from philosophy, content, style, to choreographic process, and characterized by bodily movements and rhythms — in contrast to formalized ballet. Modern dance emerged as a counterforce to the ballet, which was steeped in tradition and **codified conventions.** The early modern dance pioneers sought new forms of expression that reflected the concerns of the modern era; hence, the introduction of new costumes, the elimination of shoes, an emphasis on personal expression, more natural organic movements, and the developments of new movement philosophies. Modern dance techniques are used in many contexts.

Now that you have enrolled in your first modern dance class, which might be called something like Modern, Contemporary, Creative, Freestyle, Dance 40A, PE 5B, or movement for the theater, you may be wondering just what modern dance is. Modern dance comprises highly individualized movements, original organic movements that express the thoughtful exploration of movement preferences based upon personalized, ever-changing artistic standards. The innate nature of modern dance provides for constant redefinition of the field by practicing artists/dancers.

A Blend of Techniques   In the past, **modern dance** represented the viewpoints and movement concepts of each of several dancers or choreographers. For example, there was the particular modern dance technique of Duncan, of Graham, of Humphrey, or of Wigman. In America, two different technique concepts of modern dance were developed by two early pioneers, Doris Humphrey and Martha Graham. Humphrey identified **fall-recovery** as the falling away from and the returning to equilibrium concept. Graham identified **contraction-release** as the exhalation and inhalation, respectively, as the basis for all movement. German choreographer, Mary Wigman, whose visits to the United States had an influence on the growth of American modern dance, used the terms **die and arise,** a counterbalance between death and life. These concepts formed the basis of many of the movement concepts used in modern dance.

As the horizons of the dance artists have widened, the various movement forms have become more alike. In the past, it was easy to recognize ballet by its codified positions and movements. This is no longer true. Today many "ballet" choreographers utilize the movement concepts of the modern dancer, and many of the body placements and exercises of the ballet dancer are now used in the "modern" techniques. Many choreographers now include in their work not only the elusive modern dance techniques but also the principles of jazz and ballet, as well as adapted styles from dances of world cultures.

If the term *modern dance* is to be defined for today, it should be broad enough to include all of the diverse approaches existing now and likely to exist in the future. To continue to flourish as an art form with creative new vitality and ideas, it needs, as the dictionary states, to be modern — that is, "of the present or recent times . . . having to do with the latest styles, methods or ideas; up-to-date."

What Dance Can Do for You   Perhaps more important to you than a concise definition of what constitutes modern dance is what it can contribute to the enrichment of your life. Modern dance can help give a grace and poise to all your movements and contribute to your general sense of well-being through the pleasure of a well-toned body, increased energy and vitality, integration of mind, body, and spirit, the personal physical challenge of the dance discipline, and opportunities for self-expression. Dance can open the world of creativity and improvisation to the new dancer. It can introduce you to a new form in which you experience the joy of movement and compete solely with yourself. It can heighten your appreciation of music, the plastic arts, and all movement forms. It can increase your respect for and understanding of the dancer's profession. Also, dance can make you a better-informed audience member. And, finally, a modern dance course will expand your awareness and appreciation of the way you and others move.

DANCE AS A CAREER

Some of you may consider a career in dance as a performer or choreographer. Recent statistics indicate that many professional dancers and choreographers need to supplement their incomes by doing work other than dance, while others may choreograph, perform, and work in non-performance-related dance fields. Many people in dance are trained in more than one aspect of dance, which increases their employment chances and provides them with skills to work after the performance phase of their career winds down and opens up possibilities to share their experience and talent and develop new young dancers. Many people dance for personal satisfaction without concern for the monetary rewards. Some dancers dance for the experience and pay their bills from other sources. There is no question that one can make a living in the dance field.

Anyone who is dedicated to a dance career as a dancer must be prepared to work hard. You probably will perform before you have had five years of training, but you should continue to return to the classroom to keep your body in top condition. If you become a dancer, your body will be your working instrument, just as a violin is a violinist's instrument. Unlike the violinist, however, the dancer must build the instrument while learning technique and the skills needed to perform.

Like an Olympic athlete, the dancer should be dedicated to acquiring the greatest skill possible — not for financial gain or simply to win, but for the satisfaction of giving his or her best. No less than a devoted athlete, the dancer must be disciplined and dedicated to this high purpose.

Women have played a vital role in the development of modern dance, both as dancers and as choreographers. Men also have played an important historic role in establishing modern dance as a career option for men. Ted Shawn, along with his wife, Ruth St. Denis, established the Denishawn School and company, one of the first schools to establish the early principles of modern dance. Louis Horst, who worked as an accompanist there, encouraged Martha Graham, Doris Humphrey, and Charles Weidman to leave Denishawn. Horst served as their musical mentor and established many of the precepts of modern dance and dance composition. Paul Taylor and Merce Cunningham, principal dancers with the Graham company, established their own companies. Both choreographers continue to create innovative new modern works for their superb dancers. The Alvin Ailey Dance Company is arguably one of the most popular modern dance companies. Ailey's early work chronicled the black experience. His work is characterized by high energy, a blending of the theatrical and modern tensions, Afro-American energies, and a ballet line. His school in New York City continues to train dancers for careers in dance. In Europe, Rudolf Laban, according to critic Walter Sorell, put his stamp of genius on the development of dance in the first part of the twentieth century, comparable to ballet entrepreneur Serge Diaghilev. Two of Laban's students were Mary Wigman and Kurt Jooss, choreographer of the savage, powerful, enduring universal antiwar statement, *The Green Table*, 1932. Laban's theories continue to have an international influence on dance and movement analysis in diverse fields.

In addition to careers in performance and choreography, there are many related careers: teaching at all levels and for all ages, dance notator, reconstructor of dances, dance therapist, historian, critic, journalist, accompanist, stage technician, stage manager, video artist, dance computer specialist, multimedia performance expert, arts administrator, company manager, fund-raiser, dance publicist, dance agent, dance producer, public relations specialist, movement analysis specialist, dance medicine/science specialist, dance trainer, expert in one of the allied movement therapies (such as Pilates-based, Alexander, Feldenkrais, or Bartenieff technique), dance orthopedist, performance-stress expert, and costume, set, and/or lighting designer. This short list gives you ideas to pursue in your love for the art, as all of these specialities are necessary for modern dance to exist as a performing and developing art. Your teacher can advise you on dance career options and related interests.

Modern dance can offer a diversion or a way of life — either a brief introduction to one of the most exciting of the art forms or total dedication to a life's work. The choice is yours.

DANCE FOR VIEWING

As a dance student, you should attend dance concerts to see the finished product that was started in the studio. It is often difficult to see a live professional performance unless you live in a large city or near a university that sponsors touring companies. The alternative is to see professional performances on film and television. Many excellent films and videotapes of dance exist and can be ordered for a small fee. Commercial television seldom offers first-rate concert dance, but it does offer entertaining dance by exciting, competent performers and choreographers. Educational and public television often show new works as well as older works of leading choreographers. Many universities have fine companies or performance dance groups that offer exciting, creative productions. It is to your advantage as a student to see dance, whether good or bad. You can always learn something at a dance concert, even if it is only what not to do.

Choosing a Performance   If you live in or near an area where live professional dance performances are available, you should see as many dance performances as possible in as many different genres and styles as possible. Genres should include modern, ballet, jazz, and world dances, as well as musical theater or opera where dance is integral. You should try to see both contemporary works and works of historical significance. The more variety of dance forms you see, the greater your perspective on the larger picture of dance as a worldwide cultural activity; why people dance and what they express in their dances will become clear to you. As you see more dance performances, you can begin to discern the differences in dance forms, styles, the artistic vision of different choreographers, and the performance gifts of individual dance artists. When possible, try to see as many different dance repertory companies to observe the company style achieved by artists working together toward a common vision. You will also begin to understand the wide variety of ways dance can express the human condition. If your teacher wants you to write about a performance, check with your teacher as to what performances are acceptable for writing the assignment.

Writing about the Performance   One of the values of attending performances, evaluating what you have seen, and describing it in writing is your recognition of what is important to you, what you value, and your own process. Individual process is ongoing; it never comes to an end. Attending performances gives you an opportunity to self-evaluate, recognize your mistakes by seeing alternative solutions to movement experiences, and move forward in positive new ways. Basically, what you write about is your opinion of what you saw and what you thought about it. Give details and be specific. It might be useful to consider journalistic ideas: What happened? Who was involved? Where did it happen? When did it happen? Why did it happen? And what is your personal viewpoint on it? With experience you will learn to critique dance not superficially, but with informed opinions as a spectator of the world of dance. (See Chapter 8 for suggestions on what to look for when evaluating a dance.)

Dance Audiences   While interest in all forms of dance is rapidly growing in the United States, the audience for modern dance has traditionally been smaller than audiences for other art forms. There are several reasons for this. One is that modern dance is a relatively new art. In contrast to opera and ballet, which are often supported financially by established society, modern dance is thought by many people to exist only for the benefit of other artists and dancers. This is unfortunate. Modern dance reflects the time in which it is danced. It is usually contemporary, because it is created by and for those who are interested in the reflection of life today. Examples of modern dance works that reflect their time are Afro-American choreographer Donald McKayle's powerful classic *Rainbow Round My Shoulder,* based on the black prison gang, or Martha Graham's *Frontier,* evoking the great plains of America and the indomitable spirit of Americans.

Another reason modern dance has not enjoyed a wide following is that using the human body as a medium for art formerly carried a stigma. The Puritan influence fostered the belief that the sinful body should be hidden from view; only the mind and soul were worthy of serious study. More recently, the human body has become more acceptable as an appropriate medium for artistic expression. The belief that dancing bodies are sinful now exists only in certain sections of our society, and even there this view is changing.

Audiences and Finances

Many modern dance artists and their companies are beginning to enjoy limited financial support as they become acceptable to the general public. One artist who did a great deal to promote the acceptance of modern dance was Martha Graham. Her success came slowly and only after many years of work and dedication. She achieved her greatest success as a performer and choreographer in the late 1960s, in her seventh decade. Graham retired as a dancer in 1969 and died in 1991.

But even famous artists such as Martha Graham cannot maintain their companies on audience support alone. Most of the established professional companies are forced to rely on private foundation money or government grants. Stipulations are sometimes imposed on the person who accepts these funds. These demands may hinder or help the artist. It would be to everybody's advantage if the companies could be supported by the audiences who attend the performances.

Certainly the size of an audience is not always the best measure of the quality of a work of art. One criterion of the caliber of the artist is the ability to see new trends and to synthesize these insights in a new way. Therefore, works of art may not evoke a response from people who have not been introduced to the situation as the artist has interpreted it.

Filming and Preserving the Dance

The development of the video camera has had a profound impact on modern dance. It has made all kinds of dance easily accessible for the first time to the viewing public. Public television stations now broadcast performances of modern dance companies almost weekly to all areas of the United States. High-speed, low-light video cameras have made it easy to record all levels and forms of dance. Original works can now be preserved for viewing by later generations. Before the advent of the video camera, dance works were often performed only for a season or two and then forgotten except for still photographs and the memories of the performers and the fortunate audiences who had seen the live performances.

Notated Dance Scores

Before the advent of video cameras and playback equipment, there was no way to document dance works. Visionaries like Rudolf Laban (Kinetography Laban, 1928) and others devised notation systems to document dance since there were no video or other available resources to record dance easily. Now, in addition to the video camera and playback equipment, comprehensive dance notation systems such as

Labanotation and Benesh have been developed in the twentieth century. These systems provide a written dance symbol language that is now being used to preserve great dance works in a manner similar to that used for musical scores. The video camera records an individual performance on videotape just as music is recorded on a compact disc (CD), record, or cassette. The dance notation score preserves the dance work as near as possible to the original intent of the choreographer. Those trained in one of these notation systems can learn dances and analyze choreographic structure and style from the scores.

Sequential actions in each of the two notation examples:

- **Plié-soussou (relevé)** [Bend of the knees — spring to the balls of the feet or tips of the toes]
- **Plié-tendue side** [Bend of the knees — extension of leg to the side]
- **Plié** (second position)-**pirouette** to right [Bend of the knees — turn supported on one leg]
- **Plié-low arabesque** [Bend of the knees — extend leg to back]

Labanotation
(Arrangement notation)

Benesh
(Arrangement notation)

This book is designed to give you concrete information that will be helpful in your technique classes (Chapters 2 and 3), suggest ideas for creativity and self-expression (Chapters 6 and 7), introduce some concepts on dance evaluation (Chapter 8), review some important information on how your body moves (Chapter 4), and give you an overview of the history of modern dance (Chapter 5). Websites have been included for further information on selected subjects.

GLOSSARY

arabesque   pg. 8

codified conventions   pg. 2

contraction-release   pg. 2

die and arise   pg. 2

fall-recovery   pg. 2

modern dance   pg. 2

pirouette   pg. 8

plié   pg. 8

relevé   pg. 8

soussou   pg. 8

Chapter 2

Preparation

The human body is an instrument for the production
of art in the life of the human soul.

ALFRED NORTH WHITEHEAD

Momix Baseball. *Photo by Moses Pendleton.*

Like the centuries of dancers who have gone before, you are embarking on one of the most exciting experiences of a lifetime. Even if your dance training consists of only one course, you will be awakened to an unlimited range of body movements. You will dance about those things that concern all people everywhere — the search for an awareness of what it means to be alive, to create, and to begin to understand humankind and our place in the universe.

Having enrolled in a modern dance class, you might be asking — as many students do — a series of questions: What should I wear? How should I wear it? What happens in a dance class? How much do I need to know about music? All of these are good questions, and the answers will help you get the most out of your classroom experience.

This chapter provides general answers. To learn the special requirements of your course, check with your teacher or a representative of the class. Some teachers like to use the first class meeting as a discussion period, so you should find out in advance whether ordinary clothes or dance clothes should be worn to the first session. If you have any unanswered questions, ask them! Most teachers are used to answering questions and are happy to help. Teachers of modern dance are dedicated, knowledgeable, and creative and want you to have an inspiring experience. Questions and answers can enhance your learning.

CLOTHING

Special Requirements   Often the beginning dance student wonders why in most dance studios students are asked to wear special formfitting clothes for dance classes — clothing that could be thought of as an outer skin. There are several reasons.

Dance is a visual art that uses the dancer's body to create architectural designs in space. Any clothing that does not conform to the outline of the body will alter the designs created in that space. Another reason for special clothing is that the main concern of classroom technique is to align your body in a series of exercises that will strengthen and stretch it to make it responsive to the physical demands that will be made upon it. The teacher must be able to see the placement of your body to give an intelligent criticism of your work. Guessing what you might be doing under piles of clothing is dangerous! Faulty placement of your body in exercises will weaken and even injure you if you repeat it often enough. You could compare an overdressed dancer to a building that is covered with unnecessary exterior frills that hide its basic structure.

Dance clothing also puts you in the proper frame of mind to work in the dance class. A person usually associates certain activities with a certain kind of clothing. For example, when you swim, you wear a bathing suit. Clothing that restricts movement prevents proper exercising in the same way that ordinary clothing restricts the movement of a swimmer in the water. When you are dressed in clothes worn only while dancing, you soon associate the clothing with dancing, which, in turn, helps put you in the mood of the experience to come.

Sometimes students or their parents think the wearing of dancers' tights is immoral. Consider the clothing worn on the street today! Tights are modest by comparison. Tights, leotards, or the one-piece unitard could be compared to contemporary bicycle shorts, running tights, or ski racing pants — all appropriate to their activity.

Some teachers may require you to wear **tights** and **leotards,** others may require you to dance with bare legs, and others may allow you to wear something else — even, in some contexts, street clothing. Your teacher has a point of view intended to give you the best opportunity to fully participate in the dance experience. Dance clothing can be an especially relevant concern for many dance students, who inevitably have questions about explicitly revealing their body shapes. It may give you some comfort to know that many dance students initially feel some discomfort and self-consciousness at wearing tight-fitting dance clothing that reveals their body shapes. However, they soon learn to focus on movement rather than body shape. Ultimately, it is less about your body shape and more about your dance experience. The clothing is intended to facilitate movement and make it easier to perform and to show the visual architectural shapes you create.

Most dance schools require special clothing. This clothing can be purchased in dance specialty stores, sometimes in department stores, or through online catalog sites. Check with your teacher before purchasing dance clothing. At times your teacher may let you use knee pads for floor knee work or modern dance sandals if you have foot concerns. Usually knee pads and sandals are not necessary. Most modern dance is done with bare feet. Check with your dance teacher.

Historical Overview   Clothing worn in dance training generally reflects period, culture, and performance traditions. Historically, dance clothing has progressively become more simplified as the dance has become more physically demanding and free. In the fifteenth and sixteenth centuries, performances were conducted in halls and gardens, not in theaters proper, by amateur royal and noble performers as part of the court activity. Clothing was elaborate and expensive, and training of the courtiers in the grace of dance was conducted in daily clothing in the "gymnasium of the academic arts." When dance moved into the theaters, choreographer Jean Georges Noverre (eighteenth century) encouraged dancers to discard cumbersome garments. By the nineteenth century, ballerina Marie Taglioni dropped all weighty costumes and wore a lightweight special skirt of gauze that became the standard ballet uniform. The new garment allowed her to show her increased physical prowess. In the nineteenth and twentieth centuries, American modern dance pioneer Isadora Duncan threw off her corsets, bared her limbs, and danced barefoot. Her costumes were simple, Greek-inspired tunics and scarves. German modern dance pioneer Mary Wigman wore simple costumes based on an abstraction of Asian skirts and Asian women's trousers. Erick Hawkins, a modern dance choreographer who came from an early ballet background, eschewed the traditional tights and leotards for bare legs. In the twentieth century, the influential ballet choreographer George Balanchine used simple leotards and tights in some of his ballets, like *Agon*.

Dance clothing today reflects our time and expression, varying from the traditional to personal concepts of appropriate movement apparel. This is appropriate and in line with the tradition of the modern dance, which broke with the traditions of the ballet to pioneer a new look in dance costume as well as new ways of moving. The clothing worn by Duncan, Wigman, and Hawkins were indicative of breaking with tradition.

Women's In-Class Concerns Women usually wear tights that cover the legs and hips and a leotard under or over the tights that covers the hips and trunk. If tights are seamed, the seam is worn in the back. Panties may be worn under the tights, but under no circumstances should these garments be allowed to show. The showing of the outline of the panty beneath the leotard destroys the long look of the leg. If you feel uncomfortable without panties, perhaps a brief bikini panty will suffice. Many dancers prefer to wear a thong as an undergarment. A well-fitting bra should be worn by anyone with a breast size above 32A. Breast tissue can be torn away from the underlying musculature if the breasts are not properly supported. A sports or dance bra may be preferable to the everyday bra because it provides more support and moves easier. To avoid any punctures, the bra should not have metal clips or hooks.

With the popularization and purchase of dance wear by the general public, many styles of leotards in many new materials have become available. Likewise, clothing worn for aerobic and fitness workouts sometimes influences new dance wear. Dancers seem to delight in finding different ways to wear dance garments. The only rule to remember is that your body must be visually free and clean. Within this rule, almost anything goes.

However, be aware that loud prints or bold color combinations may not be a good idea because they can distort body line and make it difficult for the teacher to determine your correct alignment.

Men's Clothing   Men's clothing consists of tights pulled up firmly in the crotch to avoid a baggy, droopy-drawers look. The tights are usually of a heavier, less sheer material than women's tights. The seams are worn in the back. A dance belt is worn under the tights to hold the genitals firmly in place and to help prevent ruptures. The one-piece dance belt, about the same size as jockey shorts, gives more support than the athletic supporter ordinarily worn under gym clothes. Of the two belt styles available, one is similar to a formfitting swimsuit, and the other, an elastic-cloth thong style, is designed to be worn with the wide cloth part in the front. Belts are available in white, black, and suntan. The line of the belt should not show through the tights, and the belt should be the same color as the tights for the same reason.

Tights should never hang down in the crotch and distort the body line, a fault that is a clear indication of a beginning student. Male dancers frequently hold up the tights with an ordinary belt around the waist, then roll the tights down over the belt. Others hold up the tights with clip-on suspenders or with elastic bands sewn onto the tights and carried over the shoulders as regular suspenders. The suspenders give a better line in that they eliminate the bulky belt line. A tight-fitting, waist-length T-shirt or equivalent is worn over the torso. This can be tucked into the tights or can hang out if it doesn't cover the pelvic area. For both men and women, the tights and accessories should be worn so that the line of the body can be seen clearly.

Some dance schools allow dancers to wear biker shorts or leggings rather than having to invest in special clothing. The main drawback to shorts is that they do not protect your legs while you are doing floor work and do not keep the body heat concentrated in the legs, which helps keep the muscles warm. Arguably, they are not as aesthetically pleasing to the body line as tights are.

Clothing Variations   Tights and leotards are produced in many colors. Some schools insist on uniformity in the colors worn by students. Check with your teacher before buying colors other than black (worn by both men and women) or pink (customarily reserved for use by women). If you are allowed to choose your own colors, consider what colors do to the look of your body. If you want to make your body as attractive and slim-appearing as possible, black is for you. Darker colors will make you look slimmer. Lighter colors are better on a slim body. If you wear colored tights, it is preferable to wear subdued tones. Remember that bright, garish colors tend to make you look larger. The top and bottom of the outfit should blend harmoniously. A severe contrast in colors tends to chop the body visually into two sections, which is generally not flattering. Some dancers prefer to wear warm-up garments over their leotards and tights. Some teachers object to these layers of clothing because they distort the line of the body. Check with your teacher about the recommended or required clothing for your class before purchasing and wearing warm-up garments.

Care of Clothing   Dance clothing can be expensive, but it will last for years if properly cared for. Dance clothes should be laundered *after each wearing,* either in warm water alone or with soap and water, to prevent fading, rotting, and odor. Hanging all dance clothes to dry, rather than using a dryer, will help maintain their condition and original size. They should not be stored in a locker when wet with perspiration. When tights develop runs, they should be sewn as soon as practicable to ensure a longer life for them.

Showers   In addition to keeping your dance clothing laundered and fresh for each new class, a shower following a workout is good hygiene and a common courtesy to others. In some cases, you may want to shower before the class, use an antiperspirant, and if you use perfume or cologne, use it very sparingly.

PERSONAL APPEARANCE

Hairstyles   If your hair is long, it should be secured in such a way that it does not fall over your face or into your eyes. It is extremely distracting to the dancer to have hair that insists on its own creative endeavors, and it is distracting to the audience too. You should find a hairstyle that is attractive and yet practical for dance.

Accessories   Before entering the classroom, check to see if you have with you all the accessories that might be needed: extra bobby pins, elastic bands for the hair (never for the shoes, as the bands break and present a hazard to everyone working), shoes if required, notebook and pencil if requested. If you perspire heavily, a towel is a good classroom accessory. Those who wear glasses can purchase at a sporting goods store a strap to hold the glasses securely in place. Since glasses are not worn in performance, some dancers purchase contact lenses. Some teachers allow you to use knee pads. If they are allowed, it may be easier to work with a thin padding rather than with a thick one.

You should be prepared for any clothing emergency that might come up once the class work has begun. It is disturbing to the classroom continuity and to your concentration to be forced to leave the room or stop to adjust clothing. Preparation for such contingencies is the beginning of self-discipline.

Fully prepared, you put on the dance clothes and then walk into the studio to follow in the footsteps of a tradition that spans the centuries. This tradition relates to the basic needs of the primitive tribesman, the courtier of the royal courts, and even the sophisticated club dancer ecstatically moving to the pounding rhythm of the latest club music.

CLASS PROCEDURES

The Dance Studio   As you walk into the studio, you are quite likely to see a fairly large room with cylindrical wooden railings (called **barres**) attached to the walls. The dancer uses these to maintain balance while doing exercises. Some studios use a portable barre, while others do not use barres at all. In the front of the room, you might see a large mirror or series of mirrors covering one wall.

Some teachers have you face the mirror so that you can see what you are doing. Others have you face away from the mirror so that you can begin to sense what your body is doing without reliance on the mirror. Both approaches have value in your training. The first allows you to get visual feedback about your own body lines and postures. The second prepares you to become kinesthetically aware of where your body is in space.

The **sprung dance floor** is usually of hardwood designed to give slightly under the weight of the dancer's body, thereby preventing injuries and lessening fatigue. Many professional dancers refuse to dance on concrete. The floor should never be waxed or finished with a lacquer, as most gym floors are. The floor should be washed with water only — never with a cleaning agent. Soaps leave a film that makes the floor slippery. The floor should be free of splinters, nails, and small holes. Some floors are covered with a covering designed for dance, for example, Marley. To keep the floor in good shape for dance, street shoes should not be worn in the studio, as they carry street dirt onto the studio floor and may cause slick spots that could be dangerous to the dancers.

Warm-up and Cool-down   As you look around, you probably see people dressed in tights, some holding onto the barre, others seated on the floor, all warming up their bodies with simple movements before they begin more strenuous physical activity. Warm-up is probably the most important technique for a dancer to learn. It not only helps protect the body from injury but also prepares the body and the mind for the actual dance class. Although many teachers include a specific warm-up in their classes, it is your responsibility to prepare your own body for the class. All bodies are different; some take longer than others to respond to exercise and to be ready to dance.

The warm-up should start with simple exploratory movements that give you a chance to assess where you are emotionally, where you are with your body at this time, and what you need to do to get yourself ready for class. It is a chance to make the transition from your previous activities and to prepare for an interactive experience bringing body, mind, and spirit into play. You should be aware of your breath and how your breath is supporting your exploratory movements. As you work, consider what is happening **physiologically** (vital processes such as breathing), **anatomically** (body structure–movement of the skeletal parts through the joints, large arm circle), and kinesthetically (muscular sensing movement, pressing outward and pulling inward).

The method of warm-up might include

- Simple, gentle stretches (never bounce in a stretch of any kind) that help make the muscles more pliable and flexible
- A full range of movements through primary joints and interconnections of the body, such as the arms and legs and spine, to facilitate neuromuscular connections
- Movement of the large muscle areas of the body, the back and front of the body, legs and arms, to make body connectivity
- Quick walking or jogging around the studio to raise the core body temperature, increase blood circulation, and increase respiration

When you have produced a light sweat over your body, then you have prepared your body to begin to move at the level of activity your teacher may require.

The cool-down is as important at the end of a vigorous class as the warm-up is at the beginning of the class. This is a time to bring all of your systems back to normal resting positions, as well as a transition back to your routine activities. It is also a time for reflection and writing in your journal. This is the perfect time to do easy stretches in a static position, engage in slow walking around the studio, or perform movement for the entire body that is slow and sustained. You should wait until you have stopped sweating before showering and/or leaving the studio without several layers of clothing.

General Procedures   When the teacher walks into the room, he or she may be joined by a pianist or percussionist who will provide the music for the class. Other teachers use a hand drum to set the rhythm that you will dance to. Or perhaps recorded music of some kind will provide the accompaniment. The accompaniment will vary according to the individual preference of the teacher and, more often, the financial backing of the department or school. The role of the live accompanist is a vital addition to the classroom. He or she must not only be a skilled musician but also have the special skills to work with the teacher and dancers. The accompanist must keep a steady, appropriate tempo for the dancers, select appropriate music that complements the movement, and play a piece of music many times over. A good accompanist inspires dancers to move to their full potential and can be a musical resource to suggest music for dance.

The teacher calls the class members from their separate areas of the room, and thus begins your participation in the dance, which the philosopher Havelock Ellis, in *The Dance of Life,* called "the source of all the arts that express themselves in the human person." In your new adventure, you will explore the natural rhythms and physical movement possibilities of your body.

Every class has a basic rhythm or form to it. Often the class starts with the warm-up, then moves into the controlled exercises that strengthen your body and develop technique. Usually these exercises are preparing you to do some specific movements for the class on that day. Once you start the class, don't sit down, as your muscles will get "cold" and you could injure yourself. Usually the exercises become more vigorous as the class progresses. Some teachers prefer to end the class with jumps or big movements; others prefer to work the class "down" with tranquil movements so that when you leave you are not as emotionally "high."

Some teachers use the barre in their exercises; others do not. Some teachers do exercises only on the floor or standing; others rarely use the floor. All methods and approaches are valid. All teachers are working toward the same goal, which can be attained in many ways—the goal of helping you develop a beautiful and artistically expressive body.

Demonstrations   The teacher will begin the class by demonstrating movement patterns for you to follow. Some teachers may not demonstrate but rather will "talk" you through the movement. Unless the teacher specifies that you are to do the movement in your own way, try to copy the teacher's way. An important part of dance training is developing your "artistic eye" to see all the nuances of movement and then reproducing them as demonstrated. There are several reasons: correct execution of an exercise is imperative if injuries are to be avoided and physical control is to be established; mastery of the body is part of the satisfaction that comes from dancing; and those who want to be professional dancers must be able to learn movement patterns quickly and correctly. The dance world is highly competitive and without large financial resources. The choreographer who must produce a work in a limited amount of time, sometimes as little as one week, is forced to hire well-qualified, well-trained dancers who learn quickly and correctly. Dancers who can do any movement required of them by the choreographer are usually hired first. You cannot learn to dance on the job.

Improvisations   Sometimes the teacher, rather than demonstrating a movement pattern, will ask you to improvise movement. Improvisations are used for a variety of reasons. There are different improvisational structures, ranging from structured problem solving to more open structures (see Chapter 6). They may be used by your teacher in the technique class to explore nuances of a quality or concept, which can then be incorporated into a movement phrase. Improvisation fosters other beneficial expectations: it develops personal movement style in phrasing, timing, expression, and creativity; aids in intuitive, spontaneous, immediate responses to verbal and nonverbal stimuli; helps actualize inner resources and life experiences; and, among other benefits, creates group cohesion as a cooperative shared social activity. Because it does not require previous physical training in a dance technique, improvisation allows you to fully and freely move your whole body through space without the constraints of an imposed dance technique. If asked to improvise, listen carefully to the movement image given by the teacher. Don't try to intellectualize, plan the movement, or reproduce a movement that you have learned in the classroom. The chief values of improvisation are to free your body with movements that are natural to yourself, to encourage you to be spontaneous, and to stimulate your kinesthetic memory and imagination. Sometimes, to stimulate the senses or the imagination, the teacher will ask you to recall a mood, a physical or emotional state of being, or movement patterns in space and time, or to imagine how it would feel to be someone or something.

If you can allow yourself to enter into the spirit of the improvisational experience, you will find it very rewarding. It may be the area of movement where you discover whether or not you want to be a dancer, teacher, or choreographer.

Decorum   A few commonsense acts of classroom courtesy will make the class function better for all participants. Do not talk in the classroom except to ask or answer questions. To avoid accidents, be aware that you are sharing the dance studio with others. When the teacher organizes the places where you stand in the room into lines or some other arrangement, listen to the instructions. When you are asked to move across the floor, line up and wait your turn as instructed. A lot of time is wasted if the teacher has to keep answering the same questions because someone did not listen to the instructions or to an answer. Be alert and attentive — you will gain more from your dance experience.

Attendance   Students usually know how to study in a regular academic class, but many are at a loss over how to get the most out of a dance class. One of the most important things you can do is to attend every class. Reading a book, this one included, will not teach you how to dance or how to be an artist. You need the daily movement experience in order to make progress. A crash program in last-minute physical exercises before the final examination will reward you only with fatigue. If your school does not give a final movement examination, then you will probably be graded on your progress in your daily classroom work. If you are given a final movement examination, it will usually deal with the areas of movement that you have learned in class and will be evaluated according to how well you understand and execute the movements. Whether you are given an exam or graded in the class, you can take from the class only what you have gained as a person and as an artist. The pleasure of the experience and self-development should take precedence over grades, even if you are going on to graduate school.

Observing Movement   When the teacher demonstrates an exercise, watch carefully the flow of the movement and the exact positions that the whole body and individual parts of the body take in space. Next, try to move through the exercise by physical suggestion of the positions rather than an all-out physical effort. This will develop your **kinesthetic sense** or motor memory — fancy terms meaning simply the physical sensation you experience when you watch someone move, for example, in skating, dancing, falling, or jumping. Then try to do the movement as completely as possible. Watch the other dancers do the movement when you are not working, and see if they are doing the same thing the teacher did. Watch the students who move well; ask yourself why they move well and apply their approach to your own movement. Watch the students who do not move as well, and ask yourself why they are not as successful in the exercise. Observing the teacher, other students, and yourself trains your artistic eye to see the design of line, shapes, forms, and movement patterns — all elements of dance. Listen to and apply immediately the criticisms your teacher gives you, as well as those given to the class in general. The criticism is offered to help you. It is not an attack on you personally but rather a criticism to help you master technique. Your teacher is another pair of eyes working for you.

Developing a **critical artistic eye** is important to the dancer, but a word of caution is in order. Asserting that you know more than the teacher or other students is counterproductive in the classroom. Offer your opinions only when they are asked for.

Having an open mind to any and all movement is extremely important to the dancer. This presupposes a cooperative spirit with the teacher and with others in the classroom. A negative, noncooperative attitude will destroy the efforts of any teacher or fellow artist. A wise teacher — one who knows when to be firm and when to be light in approach — will encourage cooperation and a healthy climate of rapport. Good teachers recognize that intractable discipline and prodding are valid only when they benefit a potential talent. Your teacher will welcome intelligent questions and comments. You will gain the most from your classroom experience if you contribute to a spirit of cooperation and helpfulness.

Classroom Critiques Classroom feedback is a common part of the dance learning experience. Your teacher will give you or the class some kind of **critique** during the class or following the class. Comments are meant to be positive and constructive in order to help you improve in your technique, your method of learning, or your movement expression. You should listen carefully to all corrections, apply the correction immediately, remember it, and see how the correction may apply from one situation to the next. At other times, the teacher may ask the class to critique something as part of the classroom learning experience. In the technique class, comments may be

- Physical, for example, alignment
- Rhythmic, for example, starting the movement on a certain count or phrase
- Facilitative, for example, how to balance on one leg while turning
- Qualitative, for example, the kind of energy to use that will make the moves more expressive

MUSIC

In demonstrating an exercise, some teachers count out 1 2 3, 1 2 3 4, 1 2, or some other combination of numbers. Each number corresponds to a certain position that the body, or its parts, assumes in space or moves through in space. When you are asked to repeat the movement, you should attempt to arrive at these positions on the counts the teacher has indicated. The counts are then repeated in the music that accompanies the dance sequence you are doing. Some teachers "sing out" the musical pulse with sounds, words, images, or dynamic instructions to reinforce and stretch your commitment to perform and express the creative potential of the movement, not just to do a set exercise routine.

Other teachers will give you a **phrase of movement** that is to correspond to a similar musical phrase. A phrase is a certain number of counts or positions that usually make a simple statement. The movement phrase can be likened to a sentence or fragment of a sentence within the spoken language. Some teachers and choreographers work only with the musical phrase rather than with counting out the musical beats. It is probably a good idea to know how to work with beats (counts) as well as musical phrases, as both have advantages in different situations, such as in teaching or choreographing. You might try dancing to the musical beats sometimes and to the musical phrasing at other times. You will find the way that works best for you.

A few teachers prefer not to use music, phrases, or counts. They attempt to get you to move so that you sense your own movements in a prescribed or nonprescribed time. Whatever method or methods they use, you should know that dance is done in time as well as in space, and you should understand what happens when the same movements are done slowly and fast. It is important to develop your own musical sense and a feel for movement rhythm, spatial rhythm, and dynamic rhythm.

In general, rhythm has to do with the recurrence of certain elements that establish the character of the movement and movement flow. **Movement rhythm** is your own phrasing of the movements, which may or may not be performed in time to the musical structure when you are dancing to music. **Spatial rhythm** refers to the spatial patterns or pathways you establish as you move through the dance. **Dynamic rhythm** is the quality of the movement established as you use greater or lesser energy to perform a movement. Your innate or conscious choices are what make your movement unique to you and establish the style and character of your movement.

In most cases, dance is performed to music or another rhythmical accompaniment, so a basic understanding of common musical forms can be helpful. You will be expected to "keep time" with the music. Studying a musical instrument or taking a beginning course in musical theory will help your dancing by developing your musical appreciation and knowledge. You can develop your **rhythmical sense,** which will help you move in time to the beats, by listening to all kinds of music and tapping or clapping out the rhythmical pulse (beat) you feel. As an added exercise, try to analyze the structure of the musical piece. You might ask yourself such questions as how the composer has divided up the musical beats you feel, what kind of musical phrases he has used, what moods he has suggested, or what kind of transitions he has used to move from one mood to another mood. Later you might want to study specific musical forms such as the waltz, polka, or mazurka and try to identify the characteristics of these musical forms. If you like the modern sounds of the club dances, you might enjoy trying to analyze the structure of these pieces. Try to decide why this music has such a universal appeal. Is it the insistent repetition of a basic beat or the subtle, shifting rhythms? Or is it the words?

Beat   There are some basic musical structures with which all dancers work, so you should have some understanding of them. When you watch someone unconsciously tapping his foot in time with a piece of music, he usually is tapping the floor in unison with the heavy accents in the music. These are the strong beats that keep the dancers or musicians moving or playing in unison. There are also light beats (subbeats) that precede the repetitious heavy pulses in the music. A light beat occurs when the person you are watching lifts his toes from the floor. A heavy beat occurs when his toes strike the floor. (See Chapter 7 for more information regarding standard accent patterns in different meters.)

Preparation Count   Part of the pleasure of your classroom experience will be the thrill of exploring with your teacher the various rhythmical possibilities and also the qualities and forms of movement. When the teacher has demonstrated and led you through a movement combination, he or she might say something like "ready and one." "Ready" is your warning to ready yourself to move. "And" tells you to set your body in motion to move into your first position on the count of "one."

All class exercises begin with a preparation count by the teacher. This preparation count tells the accompanist and the class in what **tempo** the exercise will be danced. This tempo might be different from the one in which the exercise was demonstrated or marked. In most modern dance exercises, the count corresponds to the last few numbers of the dance phrase, cohesive movements with a clear beginning and ending. If the phrase, for example, is eight counts long, the preparation will typically be "seven and eight and." If the tempo is fast, four counts might be used: "five six seven eight." If the tempo is slow, one count may suffice: "eight and a." In all cases, the class usually remains motionless, prepared, and in the starting position of the exercise until the first beat of the initial phrase (the first "one").

Translating the rhythms and moods of the music into movements in space and time leads you toward the discipline that you must acquire if you are eventually to express to an audience your pleasure in moving. The same discipline will permit you to express your thoughts and feelings in dance. If you choose dance as a career, the discipline will help you contribute to your art as a dancer, choreographer, or teacher.

Breath Rhythm   When you are learning dance for the first time, many elements demand your attention. At times the demands can seem overwhelming, physically binding your movements so that you stop breathing and moving with natural ease. One basic element in dance that will enhance your movement and aid your freedom of movement from the beginning is learning about your own rhythm of breath inhalation and exhalation and how it supports you and the movement you are doing. As you are learning and doing new movement sequences, be aware of where your inhalation and exhalation give you a chance to exert yourself and then to recuperate from the exertion. To get a sense of breath rhythm related to movements, try these exercises: (1) widening and lengthening your body as you stretch your arms to the side while breathing in and rounding your spine and bringing your arms to your chest as you breathe out; (2) bending your knees while breathing out and straightening your knees, rising to the balls of your feet, while breathing in; (3) jumping into the air while breathing in and landing while breathing out; (4) taking three slow steps forward while breathing in and taking three quick steps backward while breathing out. What **breath rhythm** works for you? There are many elements—including breath rhythm—to be mastered in the beginning classes, but eventually your efforts will reward you with a sense of exhilaration in the sheer joy of movement and expression.

Critical Self-assessment   Your teacher is essential to your dance education, but ultimately, what you are going to get out of your dance experience will be in proportion to what you are willing to invest in it. It is useful to analyze the work of others, but it is equally useful to critically consider your own dance experiences in order to make yourself more effective in learning, performing, and creating in the dance medium. You can play a key role in your own dance education by periodically doing a self-assessment of your personal learning process. Keeping a daily or weekly journal is an excellent way to track your progress and help you understand what you are learning, what you do or do not understand, and how you can be more effective as a student. It is useful to take five or ten minutes after your dance class to write in your journal. There are many self-reflective questions you can think about, and later in your journal, you can write about those that resonate with you and your interests in the context of your own learning process.

Two important questions you might consider:

1. What observations have you made that stand out as unique and significant to you?

2. What kinds of questions would you ask yourself to make your journal and movement experience more relevant to your interests and learning process?

Other questions you might address in your journal:

3. Why are you taking this class?

4. What are your expectations?

5. Are you looking at yourself objectively, both for the positive things you are doing and for the areas in which you know you can do better?

6. What was meaningful to you in the class?

7. What was the most enjoyable part of the class?

8. What did you understand, or what needs to be clarified?

9. What did you learn: new movements, new vocabulary?

10. What questions do you have about the movements and vocabulary?

11. What was the major emphasis of the class?

12. What do you want to work on to improve your technique?

13. What is improving, and what needs more work?

14. What goals do you want to set for your next class?

15. Are you observing other students, as well as doing your best work so they can learn from you?

16. Are you genuinely receptive to new movement ideas and concepts presented in the classroom — ideas that might lead you to new perspectives and visions?

17. What practice strategy will you use at home to make the next class better?

18. What five long-term goals would you like to accomplish?

19. What has the dance experience contributed to your lifestyle choices?

20. What skills have you learned that can be applied to other classes or even a vocation?

Your best preparation for dance is your spirit, enthusiasm, and commitment. *In your journal, describe your experience, analyze it, and reflect on it.*

GLOSSARY

Chapter 3
Technique Analysis

What we do not understand, we do not possess.

GOETHE

Lar Lubovitch Dance Company, So In Love. *Photo © 1994 Lois Greenfield.*

DEVELOPMENT IN TECHNIQUE

The development of modern dance as an art form came about by the breaking of the "rules" of what dance was "supposed" to be. The traditions and techniques of modern dance continue to evolve as new gifted artists change the rules. Such change is a healthy thing. An art form can grow only when new ideas and new modes of expression come into it.

One exciting element of modern dance is the distorted use of lines, shapes, and forms to achieve a new aesthetic of beauty. Any line, any shape, any form that the human body can assume in space is valid to the modern dancer if it expresses what the dancer wants to communicate. Some beginning dancers may think the movements they are asked to do are "ugly." If you should feel that way, think of the movements as a challenge to see if you can find any similar shapes and forms in the world around you, and then try to understand their validity in an art form.

Basic Alignment   You should be aware of a few basic points about natural body **alignment** in order to understand the deviations from it. Think of your natural alignment as "good posture." Think of your body as being lengthened upward from your foot support through the top of your head. The alignment is as if you were holding onto a bar over your head and hanging down from it. Think of a straight line running down from the top of your head through your neck, torso, pelvis, and legs. This line is the central axis of your body. When you are standing, jumping, kneeling, or sitting in a good posture, be aware that your head, chest, and pelvic area stay in a straight vertical line. Your shoulders should be comfortably directed sideward and downward. Keep in mind that good posture does not mean forcing your spine to align with an absolute vertical line by straightening out the natural curves in the spine. While hanging from an imaginary string above you, allow the natural curves in the spine to happen and do not try to flatten them out.

People with bad posture may slump forward, so that their shoulders are rounded, or may release their pelvis backward, causing a swayback. Avoid both distortions of line.

The following illustrations provide a few ideas for you to consider in your basic alignment.

You should hold good alignment through various degrees of *leg rotation*. The legs can be either turned out from the hip socket or held so that the feet are pointed forward in a parallel position.

You should have *weight placement on the feet* evenly divided in a tripod between the big toe, the little toe, and the heel. When you rise to the ball of the foot (to half-toe), your weight should be between the big toe and the second toe, never toward the little toe.

Good alignment of the leg is essential to support in a *knee bend*. You should keep the center of the knee in line with the middle toe. In the small knee bend (**demi-plié**), the heels usually remain on the floor. In the deep knee bend (**grand-plié**), the heels usually leave the floor naturally, in order to prevent a pushing backward in the pelvis with a subsequent lean forward in the torso. In the turned-out side position (second position) the heels usually remain on the floor.

To *balance on one leg,* lengthen upward on the vertical line through the body. Don't "sit" into the supporting leg; that is, don't lose your pelvic support with subsequent weight shifting of the pelvis down, too far to the side, to the outside of the leg, or back onto the heel. Shift the hip toward the supporting leg and on a slight diagonal upward. In the basic balance on one leg, keep the two front pelvic bones straight across on a horizontal line.

Terminology   In general, modern dancers have not codified the terms for positions and movements. A number of modern dancers feel that codification of terms would inhibit free expression and prevent new forms of technique from developing. Another argument against codification is the infinite variety of positions the body can assume in space. Any code of modern dance movement would have to be limited and arbitrary. We have attempted to give names to body positions *only as a guide* to analyzing the infinite movement possibilities of the body. The names should be thought of as a springboard to further exploration and body analysis, not as an attempt at definitive codification.

Because different teachers and choreographers will likely use different terminology and descriptive words and imagery, you should become familiar with their working vocabulary, not only to increase your own verbal and movement vocabulary but also to make the dance experience more rewarding for you. Use of terms varies from one teacher to another. Learn the terms your own teacher uses so that upon hearing instructions you will be able to respond with the desired movement. For the purposes of analysis, definitions of basic positions are desirable. Then you as a student can both identify each basic position and understand the further development of that position. This helps you learn faster and helps train the "artistic eye" to see the subtleties of movement.

Traditional Movements   There are eight basic locomotor movements historically used in modern dance technique classes representing fundamental dance movements. Your teacher may refer to them by name or use them in various combinations. It is useful to your learning experience to be aware of various dance terms and the idea behind them. Although they are common action words, they have a specific movement connotation in dance. The eight movements are **walk, run, jump, hop, slide, skip, leap,** and **gallop.** Your teacher will guide you in the dance vocabulary he or she considers important.

FIRST ANALYSIS

Movements in a Stationary Position   While in a stationary position, you have only a few basic possibilities of movement: You can **bend** (tilt), **rotate, shift,** or **support** yourself in various ways. Despite the limited number of basic movements, however, many variations are possible, and a stationary position presents opportunities as well as restrictions. The drawings on

this page show a few of the variations. You can visualize the movement possibilities of the body by thinking of the skeleton of the body and how bony
parts are able to move through space based on various kinds of joints structured to allow for different kinds of movement. For example, the thigh
is able to move through space because
of the ball-and-socket hip **joint,** while
lower leg movement is more restricted
due to the nature of the hinge joint.

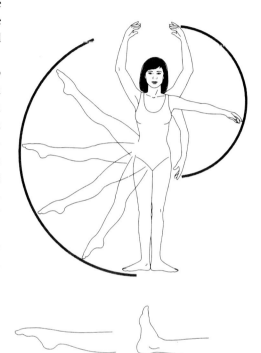

The *whole leg* can bend from the hip
socket and move in any direction, to a
certain level, with or without rotation
in the hip socket and with or without a
bend in the lower leg. The first illustration indicates various levels of the arm
and leg in the side direction. The leg
is limited in the degree of level it can
achieve, but flexibility in the shoulder
socket allows the arm to make a full circle (360 degrees), passing through the
various levels in the side direction, as
well as forward or back.

The *foot* can stretch forward to a
"pointed" foot position or bend back to
a "flexed" foot position, with or without
rotation. The *arm* and *hand* have more
freedom of movement but are similar to
the leg and foot in bending with or without rotation. The *torso* can bend in
any direction with a rounded back or straight back, to a specific level, with
or without body rotation.

The bend, or tilt, can be in the chest or pelvic area (more limited bending) or from the hip joints (greater bending). The *head-neck* can bend in
some direction that is independent of the position of the torso.

Bend (tilt)

The *torso* and its individual parts can all rotate around their own axes separately or together. The individual parts of the torso — *head, rib cage,* and *pelvis* — can do a kind of rotary action forward, backward, and sideward. The motion is more of a rocking action as opposed to the bend or tilt of those parts. The whole body can revolve completely on its own axis (turn).

The *head, shoulders, rib cage,* and *pelvis* can shift as a unit from their central **axis** in some direction.

The *body* can be supported on the floor by sitting, kneeling, lying, or standing. It can leave the support by jumping or by being lifted and held.

As a means of movement and position analysis, you could ask yourself various questions. Concerning *bending,* you could inquire: What part of the body is bending and to what level? Is the bend curved or sharply angled?

About *rotation* you could ask: What part or parts are rotated and in what direction? If the whole body is turning, is it a complete turn or only a fraction of a turn? Is the turn on one foot or both feet? What is the position of the body in the turn?

As for *shifting,* you could raise two questions: What part of the body is being displaced and in what direction? Is the shift only a basic impulse to move into another position?

And about *support* (or nonsupport) of the body, you could ask: Is a new body support achieved by jumping or rising upward to the balls of the feet? Or is it arrived at by sinking downward to small or large knee bends or positions of kneeling, sitting, or lying? What positions are moved through to arrive at the new support?

Dance is, of course, more than just stationary positions. Dance involves moving the whole body through space from one position to another. The motivation behind the movement will change the look and feel of the movement.

SECOND ANALYSIS

Body Lines   Three basic lines can be achieved in dance. These lines may be formed by parts of the body or by the dancer's entire body, as shown in the illustrations.

Vertical or
horizontal line

Oblique line

Curved line

Vertical or horizontal lines are formed when the dancer stands upright, bends at a right angle, or lies on the floor. Such lines also may be achieved in many other ways.

Oblique (slanted) lines are formed when the dancer bends at an obtuse or an acute angle in relation to either a horizontal or a vertical. Oblique lines may be formed in many ways.

Curved lines are formed in various positions. These lines may be combined with the others, just as oblique lines may be combined with horizontals or verticals or both.

Because line is so important in the dance, you should visually trace the line of movement your teacher demonstrates and try to approximate it. Sometimes you may think another line looks better or feels better for you, but remember that part of the self-discipline of learning the dance craft is to make your body do anything that choreography requires.

THIRD ANALYSIS

Feet Positions   Many modern dancers use some version of the following feet positions, with the legs either parallel or turned outward or inward from the hip sockets. The illustrations on the following page indicate the usual degree of turnout for the beginning level.

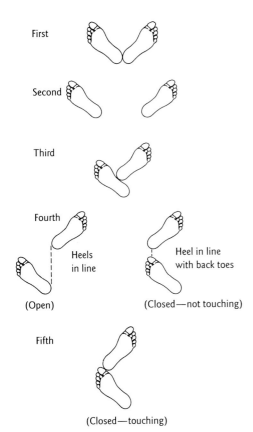

In the *first* position, the heels are together (closed).

In the *second* position, the heels are about twelve inches apart (open side).

In the *third* position (closed heel to instep), the front heel is next to the instep of the back foot, and the feet are touching.

In the *fourth* position, one foot is about twelve inches in front of the other. The heels may be in line (not crossed over), or the heel of the front foot may be in line with the toes of the back foot (crossed over—open forward-backward). This closed position is sometimes called the sixth position. Also, the open fourth can be opened to a diagonal relationship of the feet.

In the *fifth* position (closed toe-to-heel), the front heel is next to the toe of the back foot, and the feet are touching.

Following are four modifications of the first position:

The *full turnout* modification requires turnout in the hip sockets so that the toes point directly to the sides of the body.

In the *parallel* version, the legs are not turned out or in, and the toes point forward. The feet may be touching or slightly separated. Some teachers prefer that the legs be slightly separated so that the hip sockets and the bones of the legs are in a more natural alignment.

In the *diagonal-in* modification, the legs are turned in from the hip sockets so that the toes point on diagonal lines inward (this position is occasionally used in modern dance).

Body Positions   For purposes of analysis, the following definitions hold. The definitions use the basic foot positions as reference points. As the illustrations show, the definitions include various body lines, as well as movements in a stationary position.

In the *first* position, the feet and legs are together.

Standing   Sitting   Bending

In the *second* position, the feet and legs are apart to the side.

Standing   Kneeling   Bending

In the *fourth* position, the feet and legs are apart, one foot to the front and the other to the back.

Standing   Lunging   Bending in a front T

In the third or fifth position, the legs and feet cross one another in some manner (the third and fifth positions are combined here because the placement of the feet is so similar).

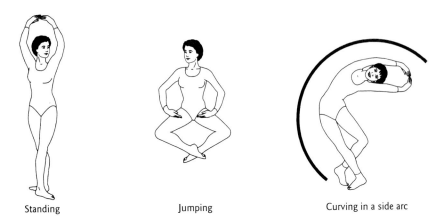

Standing   Jumping   Curving in a side arc

Arm Positions   Because the arm is more flexible than other parts of the body, more movement possibilities exist. Not all teachers will agree with the analysis that follows. Other basic arm positions may be defined. The descriptions and illustrations are presented here only as a guide to analysis. The following illustrations show curved arms.

In the *first* position, the arms are down at the sides of the body (down).

In the *second* position, the arms are raised to the sides of the body in a horizontal plane (side).

One arm is raised to the side, and the other arm is to the front—high or middle or low—in the *third* position (front-side).

First   Second   Third

The arms are in front of the body but not on the same level in the *fourth* position (front—different levels), as shown on the following page.

In the *fifth* position, shown on page 37, the arms are in front of the body and are on the same level (front—same level).

Fourth   Fifth

Examples of some variations of these arm positions follow. (With bending in the torso or rotations in the shoulder sockets, the positions also can be approximated behind the back.) These illustrations show angular arm positions, that is, the arms at sharp angles instead of gently rounded as in the previous illustrations. Here the upper arm determines the basic direction.

First   Second   Third

Fourth   Fifth

You might want to experiment, using the basic positions as a guide, to see how many variations you can discover by rotating the arms in the sockets, by changing the directions and levels of the arms, and by changing the degree of bend in the elbows.

In watching classroom demonstrations, ask the same sorts of questions that were applied to the analysis of movements in a stationary position: Are the arms straight or bent? In what direction? What is the angle of bend? Are the arms rotated inward or outward? Is the basic line curved or angular?

FOURTH ANALYSIS

Movement   Dance is, of course, more than static positions in space. Some schools simplify the analysis of movement by dividing it into two categories: **nonlocomotor movement,** which means movement around your own axis above a stationary support, and **locomotor movement,** which means movement through space to get yourself from one place to another.

In our analysis of basic movements in a stationary position—bending, rotating, shifting, and going to various support positions—we described nonlocomotor movements. However, these movements can also be done while you are moving from one place to another. Similarly, you can do many of the movements described below either while traveling in space or while remaining in one place.

Various kinds of movement analyses follow. If you imagine these kinds of movements combined into a movement sequence, you can begin to appreciate the interrelationship of your body and the space through which it moves. How the movement is done (quality or dynamics) and why the movement is done (motivation) provide infinite variations.

Descending or Rising Movement   Your body can descend toward the floor, as in a deep knee bend, or rise away from the floor, as in a jump. The individual parts of your body can also move toward or away from the floor. Falls and recovery are another common form of descending and rising. There are two basic kinds of falls. In one, you momentarily fall off balance and then quickly reestablish your equilibrium or control. Body swings from side to side are an example. In the second, you go with the natural momentum of the action until it has come to rest or until it rebounds (recovers) in another direction. For example, you fall to the floor and then rise again. Both movements are controlled partly by gravity and partly by the will of the dancer. Falls, or dropping and recovering, can be done with the whole body or with only a part of it.

Directions of Movement   The various parts of the body can move up-down, forward-backward, sideward away from or across the body, or in diagonals between front-side and back-side. And of course the whole body can also move front-back, side left or right, up-down, or on the diagonal.

An outward movement is any kind of movement that goes away from your body, as in a leg kick to the front. An inward movement is any kind of movement that comes toward the center of your body, as when you pull your outstretched arms toward your chest.

Far and Near Movements   Gestures of the arms and legs can take place away from your body, so that the emphasis may be spatially oriented. When the gestures of arms and legs take place near your body, the emphasis may be more body-oriented.

Curved and Straight Paths   The whole body or a part of the body can move through space in a curved line, that is, an arclike movement. For example, if you swing your arm in a large circle, the fingertips are tracing a circular path in space. The illustration indicates another curved pattern.

Movements can emphasize a straight line in space (spokelike) by moving toward or away from the body or by tracing a line from one point in space to another, as shown in the illustration.

Active Body   Another way of analyzing movement is to see how the body is being organized or what is emphasized. **Core-distal** movement is movement that originates from the internal muscular center outward to the extremities or from the extremities to the center. The "butterfly" in swimming is an example of a core-distal action. **Spiral** movements result when a body base is held and the free end of the body rotates, for example, facing forward and twisting the torso to see something behind you. One part of the body may be **stabilized** in order to **mobilize** another part. **Body half** movements result from stabilizing one part of the body in order to let the other body half move, for example, holding on to the barre with one hand in order to do exercises with the other half, or doing **chaîné** turns — a series of chainlike turns across the studio floor. **Upper-lower** body division might be seen in someone (upper body mobile) swinging a baseball bat to hit a ball or in someone (lower body mobile) nudging a ball forward with his foot. **Head-tail** connection relates to the integrity of the spine moving as a unified system, for example, skipping rope.

Observation and analysis of sports and daily activities are useful because each sport or daily activity, such as brushing your teeth or washing your face, requires specific body organization and movement intent in order to be successful. Successful dance techniques require a similar attention to analytical thought.

Turns   There are four kinds of turns: (1) You can twist or rotate *part of your body* on its central axis. (2) You can turn *your whole body* around by revolving to the right or left around your own central axis. There are many ways such turns can be done, for example, on your own axis on both feet, on one foot, from one foot to the other foot, or while jumping. (3) You can turn in a *traveling pattern*, for example, by walking in a circle around a chair or by doing a series of turns while traveling in a straight line. (4) The whole body (or certain parts of it) can turn, as in a somersault or cartwheel revolution or as in nodding or shaking the head. Performing various turns when sitting, lying, or supported on parts of the body other than the feet expands movement possibilities.

Locomotor Movements   Movement of the entire body in some direction through space is called *traveling*. There are many ways of traveling, and they employ the other movement patterns. The following movements could be done in place as well as traveling: (1) *walk*, (2) *run*, (3) *jump*. Jumps can be analyzed in terms of whether the jump starts from one foot or both feet and lands on one foot or both feet. There are five possibilities: from both feet to both feet, from one foot to the other foot, from one foot to the same foot, from one foot to both feet, and from both feet to one foot. The Labanotation system of analysis defines these movements, respectively, as jump, leap, hop, assemblé, and sissonne.

Whether or not these specific terms are used, recognizing the kind of preparation and landing for a jump can help you see and learn movement sequences more quickly. If you recognize, for example, that a jump starts from two feet and lands on two feet, you can quickly begin to look for other details, such as the rotation of the legs, whether the legs are straight or bent, whether the feet are pointed or flexed, and so forth.

The visual results of the walk, run, and jump will be changed by whether use of the legs is stressed or unstressed, whether there is greater or lesser use of energy to travel upward or outward through space, and the direction in which the movement travels.

Variations   Descriptions of movements sometimes used in modern dance follow. Some can be done in place, turning, or traveling. (1) *Skip* by doing a step and a hop, alternating from one foot to the other, always with uneven rhythm. The skip might also start with the hop followed by the step. (2) *Step-hop* by stepping on one foot and hopping on the same foot. The rhythm, which is usually even, may be performed even or uneven. (3) The terms *gallop,* or *slip step,* and *slide* are open to individual interpretation. Follow the interpretation of your teacher if these actions are used in the classroom. For purposes of analysis only, slide by sliding the front foot forward, transferring the weight to the front foot; then slide the back foot toward the front foot, placing the weight onto the back foot with a "cutting action" that forces the front foot to lift quickly but with very little rise and fall of the body. The gallop, or slip step, is similar to the slide except that there is a jump into the air as the weight is transferred from one foot to the other. Children demonstrate similar action when they ride an imaginary galloping horse. (4) *Prance* like a trotting horse by stepping alternately on each foot and lifting the free leg with the knee bent. (5) A *triplet* is made up of three steps on alternating feet. The knee is bent slightly on the first step, but the legs are straight on the next two steps, and the steps are on the balls of the feet. The body moves *down, up, up, down, up, up* as the knee is bent alternately on one leg and then the other. In music, a triplet is three notes that equal one quarter note. Some teachers teach the dance triplet the same way. Others treat the triplet as three steps done to three beats in the music—in other words, a waltz. (6) *Swings* can be done with individual parts of the body or with the whole body. Swings have the quality or action of the pendulum on a clock as it traces an arclike path between two points—rising, falling, rising. The rising action is increasingly sustained, and the falling action is increasingly quickened.

Body and Spatial Designs   The body, either at rest or moving, creates a form or shape in space. The body as a whole creates one kind of shape, and the spaces around the body create another kind. These shapes may be seen as straight or curved lines and are altered by the changing relationships of the body parts to one another. In symmetrical design, the body parts are equally proportioned in the space; in asymmetrical design, the body parts are not equally proportioned. The two illustrations below indicate symmetry-asymmetry and the primary-secondary design of the body and the space around it.

A second kind of spatial design can be seen by movement in opposite directions, that is, either forward-backward, sideward out–sideward across, or up-down. The direction of the movement changes the general movement shape, which can be perceived, respectively, as advancing-retreating, widening-narrowing, and rising-sinking. The illustration below suggests the movement shape of advancing-retreating.

A third kind of spatial or body design is the adaptation of the body to objects or to another person. In dance, this kind of adaptation, or sculpting of space, is often done without the presence of an actual object. The following illustration shows body adaptation in partner work.

FIFTH ANALYSIS

Qualities or Dynamics   All movement patterns take on a different look when you change their qualities or dynamics. If a pattern fails to convey some quality, it becomes devoid of any human association, and it will have little appeal to a general audience.

Qualities are related to the science of dynamics, which concerns the motion of bodies and the motivating forces. **Dynamics** is related to the greater or lesser use of energy by your body while moving in time and space. The movement may be motivated by the need to express some kind of emotional or physical state. You can use a number of basic qualities to add "shading" to your movement in the same way a painter uses contrasts in colors and shapes to enrich a painting.

The vitality of modern dance is that it is not codified. Dancers, teachers, and choreographers develop a unique working vocabulary with which students and dancers need to become familiar. The description of movement dynamics is another one of those areas. You too may add to the vocabulary. How the elements of time, tension, force, and space are combined characterize what is perceived by the viewer or experienced by the dancer as a kinesthetic experience. What follows is one perspective.

The inner motivation for the movement is elusive, but the external movement can be analyzed. For the purposes of analysis only, we have divided the qualities or dynamics into the four efforts conceptualized by Rudolf von Laban and F. C. Lawrence: **time, flow, weight,** and **space.** For each, the degree of effort used can be any point between two extremes. It is the mover's attitude toward a particular effort that determines how that person moves. In life, the kind of movement quality or effort used is in a state of flux, adapting to the internal or external needs of the moment. In dance, the dancer can consciously concentrate on changing the effort quality or qualities to add texture or shading to the movement, thereby enriching a sequence of movements. Different teachers may use their own terminology for these dynamic elements; for example, flow might be referred to as degrees of tension, weight might be referred to as force or degrees of pressure, and space might be less about the personal attitude toward space but rather how one moves through space. For Laban and Lawrence, efforts are more about the personal inner attitude that manifests itself in characteristic movement patterns. Your teacher will let you know the terminology he or she prefers.

Time   Movement may be sustained or sudden. Sustained movement can be thought of as leisurely, indulging in the use of time. Sudden movement or a series of quick motions conveys a sense of urgency.

Flow   Movement tension may be free or bound. Free flow can be thought of as unrestricted, not holding back. Bound flow can be thought of as restricted, holding back. (No negative connotation is intended by the term *bound*.)

Weight   Weight may be light or strong. Light weight can be thought of as delicate and rarefied, overcoming the pull of gravity. Strong weight can be thought of as forcefully increasing the pressure or push as the body follows the pull of gravity. (Strong weight is not synonymous with the heaviness of a person or an object.)

Space   Spatial attention may be indirect or direct. Indirect spatial attention is characterized as flexible, with many overlapping foci or many shifts of attention. Direct spatial attention is channeled into a single spatial focus. Again, it is an inner attitude toward the space, so eye contact or movement of the body may not necessarily reinforce indirect or direct attention.

Movement Exercises for Dynamics   Some movement experiments may help you sense these efforts. Suppose you were given the following movement assignments. How would you move? Do these assignments influence your attitude toward the effort quality in some way? –

Time (Sustained) Lie down on the floor and stand up as slowly as you can. (Sudden) Lie down and stand up as quickly as you can.

Flow (Free) With as little tension as possible, move about the room, freely swinging your upper body and arms. (Bound) Start to increase the tension or restrict the freedom of the movement until it feels as if you are fighting to hold back the movement.

Weight (Light) Starting curled up on the floor, unfold your body as if it were a balloon being filled with helium; let the action float you up to a standing position. (Strong) Reverse the previous action, moving from standing to curling. Get behind your weight and strongly push it downward as you lower yourself to the floor.

Space (Indirect) Move to different places in the room, rapidly changing your focus and direction. (Direct) Focus all of your attention on one place in the room and move to it directly.

All teachers are unique and have their own terms to help you understand dynamic forces and how the same movement changes when the quality is changed. Some teachers use word imagery or a descriptive phrase that suggests the quality. Examples include *protract*, prolonging the movement; *vibratory*, shaking or trembling; *percussive*, beating or striking; *suspension*, a moment when the movement is lifted and held; and so forth. Try to sense in your body the quality described and how it can alter the movement.

Emphasis in a Movement Phrase
A dance movement phrase usually has a unity or logical coherence that creates a sense of harmony or completeness, which in turn leads into the next phrase. One could think of it as a movement statement with a beginning, a development, and a transition that leads into the next statement. The next statement might be a development of the original phrase or an independent new movement statement. When music (or sound) accompanies the movement, the dance phrase may or may not accompany the musical phrase. Learning to recognize and re-create the ebb and flow of your teacher's or your own movements will bring you nearer to the goal of being able to express yourself through movement.

On page 46 are some general ideas that might aid you in analyzing what the movement phrases are about and where they are going:

1. How does the sequence start — that is, what is the first movement?

2. What is the tempo, or rate of speed?

3. Does the movement have a sense of freedom or of being held back?

4. Is there a sense of lightness, free of gravity, or does the movement suggest getting behind your weight and directing it somewhere?

5. Does the movement appear spatially focused or diffused?

6. Are the movements confined or limited to use of the space around your body, or do they use a great deal of space around the room?

7. Does the sequence of movement flow harmoniously, or is it disjointed?

8. Is the shape of the body usually symmetrical (balanced proportion of design) or asymmetrical (unbalanced proportion of design)?

9. Do the gestures and movement tend to be curved (arclike) or linear (spokelike)?

10. Is a movement accented with more force in a direction upward, downward, inward, or outward?

11. Does any movement seem to be an impulse (impelling force) leading into another movement?

12. Is there any repetitive or stressed directional movement pattern, floor pattern, or rhythmic pattern?

13. What seem to be the distinctive elements that are emphasized in the movement — rhythm, body form, line, floor pattern, or something else?

14. Can you rhythmically verbalize descriptive words that match the movement sequence, for example, slow-fast-fast-slow, up-down-out, sharp-smooth-sharp-sharp, push-pull-slash, step-step-hop, and so forth?

15. Is a characteristic manner or expression important to the movement?

16. Is there a motive or central theme that unifies the movement?

Whether or not you follow or use these kinds of dynamic analyses is not important. Modern dance grows by the diversity of approaches. What is important is developing your ability to see others' use of dynamics and to sense your own. This ability can help you learn a movement phrase — how it starts, how it develops, how it concludes, and how it makes the transition to the next phrase. By learning movement sequences dynamically, you can avoid the possibility of learning a series of disconnected steps and postures without any inherent motivating and unifying spirit. An appreciation of dynamics also allows you to begin to understand and find your own way of moving and how movement can be used for self-expression through dance—an important element of modern dance.

SIXTH ANALYSIS

Floor Patterns   Basically, floor patterns are made up of curves, straight lines, or combinations of both. Patterns may be more intricate than the paths of movement described here. Some of the basic patterns are shown below. As a means of movement exploration, try applying these basic floor patterns to movement patterns or to stationary positions of the body. (All can be done with either the whole body or parts of the body.) The arrow indicates the direction of travel, and the square represents the performance area.

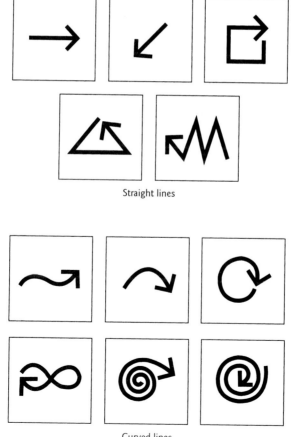

Straight lines

Curved lines

Groups of dancers also move in straight and curved lines. A few examples of floor patterns for groups follow.

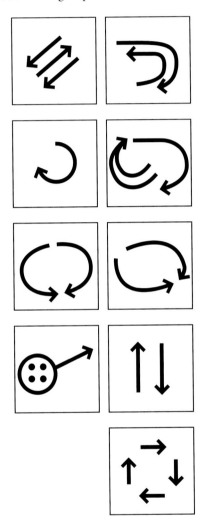

The six sets of analyses in this chapter are offered to help you more quickly learn to dance by using your mind as well as your body. Your teacher will stress some of these ideas and reject others. All approaches are valid if they help you reach your goal as a dancer.

GLOSSARY

alignment   pg. 28

axis   pg. 32

bend   pg. 30

body half   pg. 40

chaîné   pg. 40

core-distal   pg. 40

demi-plié   pg. 29

dynamics   pg. 43

flow   pg. 43

gallop   pg. 30

grand-plié   pg. 29

head-tail   pg. 40

hop   pg. 30

joint   pg. 31

jump   pg. 30

leap   pg. 30

locomotor movement   pg. 38

mobilize   pg. 40

nonlocomotor movement   pg. 38

rotate   pg. 30

run   pg. 30

shift   pg. 30

skip   pg. 30

slide   pg. 30

space   pg. 43

spiral   pg. 40

stabilized   pg. 40

support   pg. 30

time   pg. 43

upper-lower   pg. 40

walk   pg. 30

weight   pg. 43

Chapter 4

Anatomy, Injuries, and Diet

Frequently the most talented people are those most
aware of their own deficiencies and most willing to
work hard to overcome them.

LEE STRASBERG

Penrod Plastino Movement Theater, Sonata for 2. *Photo by Donald Bradburn.*

BASIC ANATOMY

Dance medicine and science, a relatively new field of study, has produced information about dancers and can give you information about your body to help you train safely, become a better dancer, and have better technique. One particularly valuable website is produced by the International Association for Dance Medicine and Science (www.iadms.org). This association offers position papers and new information about injury and training for the dancer.

It is to your advantage to be familiar with the terms your teacher uses when referring to anatomy. There are correct and incorrect ways to work your body to receive the maximum results from your effort. If you know what part of the body your teacher is talking about, you can immediately apply your anatomical knowledge to the correct execution of the exercise.

We present here only the basic anatomical facts and physiological principles from which to work. If you are interested in a more thorough study, see the excellent readings listed in the selected references.

In a single dance exercise, almost every muscle in the body is used. In Table 4.1, we have indicated only the large, main groups of **muscles** and their common functions and movements. You can dance without knowing about these muscles, but a brief introduction to them should help you understand dance movement better.

TYPES OF INJURIES

Muscle Soreness   A vigorous dance class after a period of inactivity may cause muscle soreness, which is the most common pain resulting from beginning dance classes. Such pain is referred to as **acute soreness** and will subside shortly after exercise ceases. **Delayed soreness** is another type of muscle soreness that occurs within twenty-four to forty-eight hours after exercise. This soreness, which can be severe, often increases in intensity for two to three days and then gradually subsides within seven days. A complete warm-up before dance class and a careful cool-down after class will help prevent this discomfort. A hot bath or shower may reduce muscle tension. Massage can aid the process of transmitting nutrients to the muscles. **Massage** is the healing technique that uses deep rubbing and kneading of the muscles. It is important that you use a trained, licensed professional—one who understands the dancer's body—for these services. Massage can relieve muscle tension, edema (fluid buildup in tissues), and soreness.

TABLE 4.1   Movements and Functions of Main Muscle Groups

Parts of Body	Main Muscles	Approximate Location	Main Movement
	Biceps	Top of upper arm (when arm is lifted to side at right angle to body with palm up)	Bend or flex elbow
	Triceps	Bottom of upper arm (when arm is lifted to side at right angle to body with palm up)	Straighten or extend elbow
	Pectorals	Front of chest	Bring arm across chest, lower arm when overhead
	Trapezius and latissimus dorsi	Upper back Middle back	1. Move scapulae 2. Pull arms downward, backward, and inward
	Obliques	Over ribs on either side	Twist upper body to either side
	Rectus abdominis	From upper ribs to top of pubic bone, covering abdominal area	Raise upper body forward as in sit-up
	Quadratus lumborum	Small of back	1. Bend upper body to side 2. Stabilize pelvis and spine
	Iliopsoas	Lumbar spine to femur	1. Strong hip flexor 2. Raise thigh to trunk *or* flex trunk to thighs against resistance
	Gluteals	Buttocks	1. Stabilize hip 2. Extend hip
	Quadriceps	Front of thigh	Extend leg in forward movements
	Hamstrings	Back of upper leg	1. Bend knee 2. Extend hip
	Gastrocnemius (gastrox or calf)	Back of lower leg	1. Point foot 2. Raise leg to ball of foot (half-toe) 3. Bend knee
	Tibialis anterior	Front of lower leg	Flex foot (dorsi-flexion)
	Tibialis posterior and peroneals	Around either side of ankle	All muscles contribute to move ankle in circle
	Achilles tendon	Lower part of leg and heel on back of leg; longer part of gastrox (calf) muscle	Same as gastrox

Common Exercise and/or Weight-Training Suggestion	Significance for Dance	Discussion
Push-up and pull-up Weights: curls (bending the lower arm to the upper arm while holding weight)	Strengthens arms for falls and lifts	Generally very weak in women; both men and women need this strength for control
Push-up Weights: standing triceps extension; hold weight in both hands overhead, lower weight to neck level and to the back and up again	1. Strengthens arms for falls and lifts 2. Gives firmness under the arm	Development imperative for control of back and upper arm strength
Push-up Weights: Bench press, dumbbell fly, and pullover	1. Provides firm chest muscles 2. Needed for lifts and falls	Strength needed for development of chest
Push-up, pull-up, chin-ups Weights: with arms extended wide apart overhead, pull weight down to neck level and push back up	Gives control of entire back and arms	Development of entire back for control in balancing off-center turns and body control in general
Twist or rotate upper body	Makes small, strong waist	Vulnerable in lifts; can be strained
Sit-up: with knees bent and legs at 90°, crunch or raise only upper body toward knees	Keeps abdomen flat if done regularly	Strength of this area increased by twisting movements during sit-up
1. Bend upper body to side 2. Sit-up as described above	Contributes to strong lower back	*Injury*—General weakness; sit-ups and stretches of the back imperative
Stretch the thigh to the back while maintaining the integrity of the hip	Can contribute to lordosis or swayback	Must be stretched constantly
1. Turn out leg from hip socket 2. Lift leg to back 3. Weights: leg press	Contributes to thigh turnout	Must be developed in males, especially for strength in leaps and jumps
1. Lift leg forward 2. Straighten leg at knee joint 3. Pull up kneecap 4. Weights: quadriceps press	1. Steadies knee joint 2. Straightens knee 3. Provides stability for knee joint	*Injury*—Strain At onset of pain, apply ice; rest until pain stops; do easy movements
1. Touch toes with fingers without bending knees 2. Sit erect on floor with legs extended straight forward 3. Weights	1. Bends knee 2. Must be stretched constantly and also strengthened	*Injury*—Strain At onset of pain, apply ice; rest until pain stops; no stretching until no pain. Strengthening is often neglected in dancers.
1. Jump 2. While holding weight, rise up and down on a raised surface so heel drops below surface	1. Tires easily 2. Strain muscle in jump 3. Points ankle and foot (plantar flex)	*Injury*—Temporary soreness from sudden overuse and strains *Prevention*—Should be stretched more
Overuse common Do toe pulls with towel	Flexes foot and ankle	Major part of shin-splint syndrome. Ice, stretch board needed
1. Rotate ankle in circle 2. Raise and lower on stair or board	1. Helps protect Achilles tendon 2. Supports ankle in all foot movements	*Injury*—Sprained ankle *Prevention*—Keep ankle in line with center of knee
Jump Weights: calf machine	1. Must be stretched constantly 2. Thickest and strongest tendon in body	*Injury*—Tears apart by violent overstretching *Prevention*—When coming down from a jump, land on ball of foot, lower heel to floor, bend leg

Pain from Injuries   Pain resulting from an injury is an entirely different feeling, and proper care of the injured part must be administered in order to prevent possible permanent damage. For the most part, an injury occurs when a part of your body is weak and/or when you are tired either physically, psychologically, or both. Other reasons for dance injury include postural malalignment, repetitive dance techniques, falling, tripping, sudden very quick movement, accidental contact with other dancers or objects, nonsprung floors, a cold environment, lack of warm-up, and failure to rehabilitate an existing or old injury. In any class, if you are in good condition and if you work correctly, injuries should rarely occur.

Cramp   A common pain is the **cramp.** A muscle cramp occurs for many reasons, and researchers do not agree on the cause. Some believe cramps occur through a problem with the mechanism that controls a muscle contraction. Others believe inadequate stretching, lack of warm-up, and/or muscle fatigue may contribute to cramps. Other factors may include dancing in extreme heat, dehydration, and depletion of electrolytes. A cramp usually occurs in the arch of the foot or the calf of the leg. The pain occurs because the muscle goes into a maximum contraction involuntarily. To relieve a cramp, stretch the cramped part very gently or massage it in order to get a fresh blood supply to it. Generally, no permanent damage results from a cramp, but the muscle may be sore. Usually you may continue dancing as soon as severe pain subsides. Drinking lots of fluids may help prevent cramps.

Skeletal Injuries   We can discuss only a few of the more prevalent skeletal injuries that dancers experience. General care of such injuries must include rest, ice, compression, and elevation (**RICE**). Ice or cold compresses must be applied immediately after an injury. This helps reduce the swelling, thereby reducing pain. You must inform your teacher as soon as any type of injury occurs. Any *major* injury must be seen by a health professional as soon as possible. This may be the school nurse, the athletic or dance trainer, or a physician. You or a friend should not try to diagnose your injury. It is hoped that dancers have access to the athletic trainer for help with injuries, as he or she is a part of the staff in most high schools and institutions of higher education.

Sprain   A **sprain** occurs when a joint goes beyond its normal range of movement and ligaments are damaged. This injury does not heal easily and demands a doctor's care. Ligaments and capsules in the hip and shoulder may be injured in this manner, but more commonly the injury takes place in the ligaments of the ankle. It is imperative that ice or cold compresses be applied to the area until a doctor can be consulted.

To prevent a sprained ankle, it is extremely important that the knee be centered over the ankle at all times, especially when landing from a jump or leap. If you are prone to a sprain in any part of your body, consult your doctor or teacher for exercises to strengthen that area.

Strain   A **strain** is usually caused by inadequate warm-up or poor flexibility. It usually occurs in the quadriceps (front of thigh) or hamstring (back of thigh). This pain can be relieved by ice and rest. Strains rarely result from taking just one class.

Shin Splint   A more serious injury is the **shin splint,** which afflicts the muscles on the front of the tibia (shinbone). The name shin splint is given to a myriad of complicated injuries to the lower leg that demand the care of a health professional. Extreme severity of this syndrome can lead to stress fractures, so it is imperative that the dancer be treated immediately when symptoms appear. Shin splint injuries are characterized by pain and irritation on the front of the lower leg. Ice, rest, and working on a stretch board sometimes help relieve these symptoms.

Many other kinds of injuries could occur in a dance class, but if you work properly, injuries should not occur.

INJURY PREVENTION AND RECUPERATION

The training of a modern dancer has continued to change since modern dance as an art form began. Current training methods reflect the increasing demands of more difficult techniques and higher performance standards. Although these rigorous criteria have produced more injuries, health professionals, dance teachers, and choreographers are now more conscious of how to care for dancers so that injuries don't occur. Only recently has the public become aware of the injuries faced by dancers and that a dancer is one of the finest-trained athletes.

A twenty-year study by the Dance Medicine Group at the authors' university (University of California, Irvine) on the physical screening and follow-up of over 1,000 student dancers has shown that the majority of injuries in student dancers occur from the hip down. This same incidence has also been reported in the literature on professional dancers. Recently, we have seen an increase in upper-body injuries, which seem to come from the new demands of choreography. Many choreographers now invent movements that demand greater upper-body, shoulder, arm, and wrist strength than had been required in past years.

Although a dancer can sustain a sudden sprain, strain, or break, the most common injury develops over a period of time through overuse. The continual repetition of the same movements causes most of the injuries in dance. High-level student and professional dancers experience these overuse injuries more often than do beginning or intermediate student dancers, because professionals and many dance students dance at least eight hours a day six days a week.

Your schedule as a beginning or intermediate student usually includes one or two dance classes a day and perhaps two or three additional hours a week in rehearsal. Performances are usually scattered throughout the year. This schedule should not produce injuries that keep you from dancing, but it may produce problems in your body similar to those problems the professionals have, because you also perform the same kinds of movement over and over again.

Most of the injuries you will incur involve the **soft tissues:** muscles, tendons, ligaments, and bursae. These are acute injuries, which means that you must rest the area of the body that hurts. To stay in shape during your recuperation, you should do other types of exercise that do not involve the injured part.

Exercise   We recommend several forms of exercise to increase your strength and endurance, both when you are healthy and dancing and when you are recuperating from an injury. An additional problem with any injury is the possibility of its recurrence. This is why alternate and additional forms of conditioning, such as weight training, warming up, and cooling down, are so important to the continued health of the dancer. There are other ways to condition the body, including Alexander and Feldenkrais techniques. Frederick Matthias Alexander created an integration of movement for the body to eliminate tension and improve posture. He based his system on the positions and placement of the head and neck. Moshe Feldenkrais based his system on doing small movements with full awareness. He felt all movement should focus on the skeletal system, not the muscles, and that movement should be done with maximum efficiency and grace. Other forms of conditioning include low-impact aerobic exercise designed especially for the dancer, water exercises, Gyrotonics imagery, stationary bicycling, and Pilates-based exercises—but they are too detailed to include in this book. Any additional conditioning program *must* be discussed with and approved by your teacher so that the extra work enhances your performance and does not damage it.

Weight Training   We have chosen to discuss weight training as a form of additional conditioning for dancers for two reasons: (1) it is the most readily available form of conditioning, since most schools and all private health clubs have the equipment, and (2) the authors have had remarkable positive results from the weight-training program in their own department over the past ten years. New information indicates that weight training for female dancers must be accomplished with high weight and low repetition to build strength without bulk. A female dancer should use a sufficient amount of weight to stress the muscle but not so heavy a weight as to fatigue the muscle too quickly. It is important to train both the lower and upper body and to perform all the movements through a full range of motion. Dancers will not lose flexibility when lifting weights if they warm up before lifting and continue to take their regular dance classes. Male dancers need to do the more traditional weight-training protocol that particularly develops the upper body and also includes work on the lower body. We recommend that both male and female dancers lift weights three times a week.

No dancer should begin to lift weights without instruction from a weight-training coach; most educational institutions have such an expert on staff who will provide the necessary instruction. As an incentive to start a weight-training program, you should know that almost all Russian male ballet dancers lift weights and that the women and men in many modern-dance companies in the United States participate in conditioning exercises, including weight lifting.

Proper Body Alignment   Prevention of injury is best accomplished through correct alignment and proper working in class, rehearsal, performance, and the off-season, which is often the summer months for students. Many injuries that do occur in dancers can be directly related to faulty technique and incorrect placement of the body. We discussed basic alignment in Chapter 3; we now show the placement of the body as viewed from the side with the plumb line in order to reinforce the importance of proper body alignment. It is, of course, even more important that the body be properly placed when moving in dance. Your teacher is the expert who can tell you when you are "out of alignment." Some of the more prevalent alignment problems that may cause later injuries include hyperextended knees (swaybacked knees), lordosis of back (swayback), pronation of feet (roll-in), supination of feet (roll-out), and knock-knees. You should be aware of these basic common discrepancies in body alignment so that you can avoid or correct them.

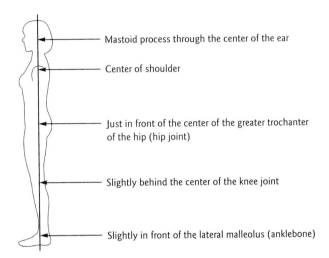

Mastoid process through the center of the ear

Center of shoulder

Just in front of the center of the greater trochanter of the hip (hip joint)

Slightly behind the center of the knee joint

Slightly in front of the lateral malleolus (anklebone)

Dancers are slightly more forward in their posture than nondancers, because they must be ready to rise to their toes or to move quickly and in any direction at any moment. This is why proper alignment is so important.

Warm-up and Cool-down   **Warm-up** serves two main functions for dancers: (1) it brings focus to the body and the mind for the important work ahead, and (2) it prepares the physical instrument to perform those functions by raising the core temperature of the body. Every dance class must be preceded by a warm-up period. A general warm-up should last from eight to ten minutes and engage the major joints and muscles. The warm-up should start slowly and gradually add increasingly difficult movement. Advanced range of motion should be increased only after the joints are pliable and the body is sweating. Research has shown that the warm-up should occur no more than fifteen minutes before a perform- ance. **Cool-down** is as important as warm-up and must occur after every class and performance. This is the time to let the heart rate return to nor- mal (about 100 beats per minute), do stretching exercises, and let sweating subside. Usually, five to ten minutes after a class is adequate time for the body to cool down. Fewer injuries seem to occur in those dancers who warm up and cool down.

Proper Rest   Getting proper rest is one of the most important ways to prevent injuries. Many times, injuries occur because the dancer is ex- hausted either physically or psychologically, or both. You probably will be working or going to school full time in addition to studying dance. With this double burden, you must establish your priorities in a way that enables you to rest and to get the sleep you need.

DIET AND FITNESS

Modern dance should not produce the bulky muscles familiar to a football player or a wrestler. These sport activities warrant the development of heavy muscles for strength. As a dancer you need long, lean lines so the clarity of the movement is not obscured. You need minimum weight so you can perform intricate movements easily.

You as a dancer must convey the ideal physique or figure. No one has a perfect body! But by proper dance training and a proper balance of exercise, rest, and diet, you can more quickly achieve the illusion of the ideal.

Dancers are notoriously abusive of their bodies. They often expect their bodies to respond instantly and perfectly on command without having given them proper care. You cannot expect to deal with the great physical demands made on your body without properly caring for it.

The word *diet* often suggests hunger, regimented eating, or eating only certain kinds of foods for extended periods. To the dancer, *diet* should signify temperance in living habits.

As a dancer, you cannot afford extra calories in foods that do not make an appreciable contribution to your body. Even if you are of a good weight, size, and structure to be a dancer, it is to your advantage to evaluate your daily intake of food.

The current dietary recommendation for active teenagers and young adults is to choose foods from all food groups, following the 3-4-4-2 dietary plan each day. This translates to 3 servings from milk and milk products, 4 from vegetables and fruits, 4 from grain products, and 2 from meats and meat alternatives. Athletes often follow a different dietary plan, which combines the meat and dairy groups to compose one group of foods. They consume the bulk of their diet from the vegetable/fruit and grain groups. The ideal dietary plan for dancers is 60 to 70 percent complex carbohydrates (sugars and starches), 15 to 20 percent fat, and 15 to 20 percent protein to produce abundant energy.

Either dietary plan can work for you. The key fact to remember is that one gram of fat contains nine calories, whereas one gram of carbohydrate or protein contains four calories. You can, therefore, eat more carbohydrates or protein and consume fewer calories than you would with the same amount of fat.

To explain the physiology of the energy cycle in simple terms, we begin with complex carbohydrates, which are stored in the body as glycogen.

Glycogen is broken down into **glucose,** which is the main fuel for muscular activity. Glycogen is not easily stored in the body; this is why carbohydrates must be continually replenished. Dancers do not use as much energy as do endurance athletes, so they usually need fewer calories.

The importance of a balanced diet during the adolescent and young adult years cannot be overemphasized, especially for active dancers. Adequate vitamins, minerals, and calories must be consumed to keep you healthy now and to prepare your body for the later years. Female dancers need to be especially concerned with consuming adequate calcium (nonfat milk and milk products, tofu, greens, legumes) and iron (red meat, eggs, green vegetables, legumes). Vitamin and mineral tablets have sometimes been recommended to supplement this part of the diet. Supplements must be taken in conjunction with the proper foods in order to be fully beneficial. Taking them is not recommended unless you are directed to do so by a physician or registered dietitian.

If you want to lose weight, you should be able to do so on 1,500 calories a day (we do not recommend fewer calories than this), especially if you are taking dance classes at the same time. If you do not lose weight, you may have a medical problem. See your physician if this situation occurs.

The reduction of fat in your diet and the addition of carbohydrates, especially fruits and vegetables, will help you lose weight and hopefully gain more energy. Fat comes mostly from butter, whole milk, cream, untrimmed meats, and the unsaturated vegetable oils that are in margarine and most foods stored on the grocery shelf and sold in fast-food establishments. Lean beef, skinless poultry, and fish are almost entirely protein, and complex carbohydrates come from whole-grain cereals and breads, pastas, fruits, and vegetables. Of course, several foods, such as legumes (peas and beans), have both protein and carbohydrates.

Here are some ways for dancers to lose or maintain weight:

1. "Grazing" (eating several small meals daily) is an especially effective eating regimen to accommodate the intermittent schedules of students and performers.

2. Coffee, tea, and diet colas have zero calories, but the caffeine in these drinks dehydrates and stimulates the body when your body is actually in need of rehydration (fluid). Water is the best fluid for all dancers. Try to drink eight glasses of water every day.

3. Eat fruit, raw vegetables, yogurt, and air-popped popcorn in place of cookies, chips, and salty snack foods.

4. For dessert, eat nonfat frozen yogurt; one cup has only 144 calories, compared to 349 calories or more for one cup of ice cream.

5. Participate in an aerobic activity for thirty minutes, three times a week. This includes swimming laps, running, taking fitness classes, riding a bicycle, using a treadmill, or engaging in other physical activities.

6. Establish a reasonable weight-loss goal of no more than one pound a week, and do not weigh in more than once a week. Remember that it takes a long time to gain weight, and it takes the same amount of time to lose it. Try to be reasonable. See "Nutrition Fact Sheet: Fueling the Dancer," by Priscilla Clarkson, Ph.D., and presented by the International Association for Dance Medicine and Science on their website (www.iadms.org).

The preoccupation with abnormal thinness that now permeates our society has produced an alarming number of sufferers from eating disorders. These disorders are not limited to professional and student dancers; it is now believed that more than 20 percent of young women suffer from more than one of the symptoms of an eating disorder. But we do know that the extreme thinness expected of dancers, gymnasts, models, and some other female athletes has made eating disorders a reality in these groups as well as among male wrestlers and jockeys, who must "make weight," and male divers and models, who also rely on the "look of the body to perform the skill."

There are two types of eating disorders: **anorexia nervosa,** or self-starvation, and **bulimia,** a related syndrome involving binge eating followed by vomiting, laxative abuse, use of diuretics, or fasting. Both disorders can be fatal if carried to extremes, so it is imperative for a person who suffers from either of these disorders to seek help as soon as possible. Some of the symptoms of eating disorders are low self-esteem, guilt when eating high-calorie food, obsessive preoccupation with weight, and unrealistically high goals and expectations of oneself. Often another dancer or a friend can identify the problem before the teacher becomes aware of the situation. It is important that you talk to your teacher confidentially about the possibility of you or anyone you know having an eating disorder.

Avoiding injuries, maintaining leanness, and giving maximum energy are the major concerns for dancers. Understanding the body and how it functions contributes to the essence of a dancer's existence.

GLOSSARY

acute soreness   pg. 51

anorexia nervosa   pg. 61

bulimia   pg. 61

Chapter 5

History

For last year's words belong to last year's language
And next year's words await another voice.

T. S. ELIOT

Lewitzky Dance Company, Episode #1. *Photo by Vic Luke.*

extraordinary illusions. She was hailed as an original movement artist at the turn of the century, at about the time of Duncan. She had a great following and reputation in France, which was the center of much of the expressionist movement at the turn of the century. The United States, her birth land, did not give her a warm welcome. She helped Isadora Duncan organize her first tours of Europe.

Duncan's search for a natural movement form sent her to nature. She believed movement should be as natural as the swaying of trees and the rolling waves of the sea and should be in harmony with the movements of the earth. These beautiful ideals have often been misinterpreted and grossly misused in dance. Modern dance has often been thought of as young girls imitating the blooming of a flower. Contrary to popular belief, Duncan never improvised on stage and personally supervised every detail of her performances. Her great contributions are found in three areas.

First, she began the expansion of the kinds of movements that could be used in dance. Before Duncan danced, ballet was usually the dance performed in theater venues. In the ballet, the feet and legs were emphasized, with virtuosity shown by complicated, codified positions and movements. Duncan performed dance by using her entire body in the freest possible way, taking her inspiration from the ancient Greeks. She did not develop a technique as we know it today. Her dance stemmed from her soul and spirit. She was one of the pioneers who broke tradition so that others might be able to develop the art.

Her second contribution was in dance costume. She discarded corsets, ballet shoes, and stiff costumes and replaced them with flowing Grecian tunics, bare feet, and unbound hair. She believed in the natural body being allowed to move freely, and her dress displayed this ideal.

Her third contribution was in the use of music. In her performances, she used the symphonies of great masters, including Beethoven and Wagner, which was not the usual custom. Other dancers had used this music, but Duncan made it popular with the large audiences that admired her dancing.

She was as exciting and eccentric in her personal life as in her dance. She threw away the conventions that characterized the time in which she lived. She has been portrayed in a film, *The Loves of Isadora,* and the dancing in this film is a near duplication of the way Duncan moved.

Whereas Isadora Duncan looked to the West and to classical Greece for inspiration for her new dance, Ruth St. Denis (1877–1968) looked to the East and the Orient to discover a new movement form. In 1906, she performed *Radha,* a dance that used an Oriental theme to communicate a spiritual message. It was so significant that it continued to be performed even in the 1940s, when Miss Ruth (as she was usually addressed) was in her sixties. She was interested not just in virtuosity in dance but also in communicating an idea. She did not develop a technique. Instead, she believed music was to be "visualized" in order to produce dance movements.

In the scheme of the development of modern dance, Ruth St. Denis holds a vital position. She not only made specific contributions of her own but also provided, through the Denishawn Company, a proving ground for the next generation of dancers, including Martha Graham, Doris Humphrey, and Charles Weidman. Denishawn, which was a partnership and a marriage between Miss Ruth and Ted Shawn, proved successful for some sixteen years. During these years, Denishawn was financially self-supporting—a unique position in the history of modern dance companies.

Ted Shawn was codirector of Denishawn, and if Miss Ruth was its spirit, he was its form. He performed and choreographed in Denishawn until it dissolved in 1931. From 1933 to 1940, he directed a company of male dancers who were ex-athletes. He was influenced by François Delsarte, who in the early nineteenth century had developed a technique of pantomime that honestly expressed emotion. Shawn wrote about these techniques in a book, *Every Little Movement.*

Shawn taught baseball, football, and basketball players, wrestlers, and track stars dances with strong masculine themes, such as *Olympiad* and *Labor Symphony.* Through his efforts, he helped raise the status of the male dancer in the United States by choreographing themes that promoted the masculine characteristics of the dancers.

Another major contribution by Ted Shawn to the dance world was the founding of the Jacob's Pillow center in Massachusetts. This is a residence for dancers where they may study and perform. Late each summer, a festival is held there where works are presented in concert.

Mary Wigman (1886–1973), who came from the German School of modern dance, was another influential pioneer. Wigman was regarded as the genius and the leader of German modern dance from 1924 to 1943. She studied dance with Émile Jacques-Dalcroze (1865–1950), who created a way to teach the coordination of music and body movements called **eurythmics,** and with Rudolf von Laban, who developed one of the methods of recording body movements on paper, which is now called **Labanotation.**

Because she was concerned with self-expression, Wigman's contributions included psychological and emotional approaches to creativity. She felt that dance should be movement alone, so she composed dances without music. She fully explored the use of space. Her dances were described as "dark and somber . . . largely an ecstasy of gloom, stressing the demonic and macabre" (Margaret Lloyd, *The Borzoi Book of Modern Dance* [Brooklyn: Dance Horizons, Inc., 1949], 12).

Ruth St. Denis

Martha Graham

Merce Cunningham

Doris Humphrey, Charles Weidman

Mary Wigman

Ted Shawn

Bella Lewitzky

Alvin Ailey

Alwin Nikolais

Isadora Duncan

Hanya Holm (1898–1992), Wigman's pupil, adapted the German modern dance to the needs and characteristics of American dancers. As a master teacher of modern dance, she influenced many dancers with her concepts of space. Holm was one of the few modern-dance choreographers also successful as a choreographer for the Broadway musical stage. Her most famous musical was *My Fair Lady.*

Probably the most exacting technique and the greatest number of choreographic works have come from Martha Graham (1894–1991). Her technique is built on the breathing cycle of the body and its principle of "contraction and release." (Other principles developed by her are "motor memory" and "percussive movement.") In brief, Graham's dance is built on the process of inhaling and exhaling. She believed that in inhaling, the body has an aerial quality of release, and in exhaling, the body "drive has gone down and out" in contraction. Many of today's dancers, choreographers, and modern dance classes have been influenced by her technique.

Another major contribution by Graham has been in the area of choreography and performance. She is considered to have been one of the finest dance concert performers. She utilized the wide spectrum of life in the themes of her outstanding works. She often used themes from Greek drama to symbolize and probe humans' inner qualities. Her dance company has included some of the outstanding dancers in the world.

Martha Graham was a member of the Denishawn Company and a protégée of Ted Shawn. She left the company in the mid-1920s to form her own group. Both Graham and Doris Humphrey developed theories and philosophies of movement that are significant to the growth of modern dance, and both are considered to be in the art's third generation (see the Modern Dance Family Tree).

Doris Humphrey (1895–1958) was a protégée of Ruth St. Denis, and her movements were of the same lyrical quality. She also left Denishawn to form her own company, and she built her dance principles on the "fall-recovery" theory, which she created. She believed dance movement came about by periods of unbalance and balance in the body. She stated that fall-recovery consisted of three separate movements: the *fall,* the *recovery* from the fall, and the *suspension* held at the peak of recovery. She also perfected compositions using large-scale dramatic themes for groups of dancers.

Humphrey formed an alliance with Charles Weidman (1901–1975) after leaving Denishawn. Weidman had also been in the Denishawn Company and was known for his biting, satirical dance works and for his skill as a performer. Together they formed one branch of American modern dance. Humphrey performed her works until 1945, when crippling arthritis ended her performing career. She continued choreographing and working until her death.

Some of Humphrey's most brilliant works from 1945 on were created for José Limón (1908–1972), an important choreographer in his own right. His powerful body and magnificent carriage and bearing always marked his strong masculine performances. Limón formed his own company in 1946 and continued to choreograph dramatic works until his death. His company continues today under the direction of Carla Maxwell.

Lester Horton (1906–1953) was a major modern dance teacher and choreographer who chose to work in Southern California rather than New York. His dance technique is one of the three to survive from those of the early modern dance pioneers (see the Modern Dance Family Tree). Graham's and Humphrey's are the other two technique forms widely taught today. Horton was known for his use of form and color, the theatricalization of ethnic dance forms, and the development and training of other significant artists of modern dance. Some of those artists include Alvin Ailey, Carmen DeLavallade, James Truitte, fashion designer Rudi Gernreich, and Bella Lewitzky.

SUCCEEDING GENERATIONS OF MODERN DANCERS

Dancers Who Studied with Graham, Humphrey, and Horton   Of the dancers who worked in the 1960s, Merce Cunningham (1919–) has stirred the most controversy with his works. Cunningham choreographs "by chance," holding to the idea that "any movement can follow any other movement." Regarded as avant-garde, he choreographs and performs works that audiences either adore or abhor, depending on their individual convictions. His admirers point to his fine artistic sense, his intelligence, and his superb company as factors that make the works he creates brilliant movement pieces. He has often included the works of other artists (Andy Warhol and Robert Rauschenberg) in his dances. He is known for his use of video and digital technologies to enhance his works, and he continues to explore new ways of creating visual pieces using dance and technology. Cunningham maintained a long artistic collaboration with composer John Cage (1912–1992), known for his philosophy that all sound should be regarded as music. Works produced under their collaboration created new artistic realms.

Alwin Nikolais (1910–1993) has been recognized as one of the most innovative choreographers of the twentieth century. His contribution was in the creation of a form of theater that includes props, costumes, films, slides, sound, and light as extensions of the bodies of the dancers. His visual effects and illusions often remind the audience of events in their own experience, yet the works contain no story or conventional plot. The dancers' bodies are often distorted or hidden in the costumes and props to emphasize Nikolais's abstract images and suggestions. Murray Louis (1927–) danced for and collaborated with Nikolais starting in 1949 and continues to challenge the dance world with new directions.

Anna Sokolow (1910–2000) was another renowned choreographer, whose powerful social statements characterized her works. Her commitment to the socialist movement, evident in her early works in the 1930s and 1940s, gave way over time to a more general concern about the feelings and problems of all humanity. Sokolow used many different types of music, including jazz, and choreographed extensively in Mexico and Israel, as well as in the United States.

African American Choreographers   Many modern dancers have contributed to the development of modern dance as an art in America. Alvin Ailey's (1931–1989) great gift was his ability to present exciting theatrical pieces that reflect the black experience. His first company (1958) was composed of all black dancers, but now his company comprises dancers of all races who perform works by many choreographers. The present Alvin Ailey repertory company performs works that combine art and a unique vision of dance. The company is very popular and tours regularly. Judith Jamison (1943–) currently directs and creates new works for the company.

Several other black dancers have significantly influenced modern dance. Donald McKayle (1930–) is known for his use of dramatic tension and narrative to portray the black experience in his dances. One of his best-known works is *Games*, which is based on children playing in the city streets. McKayle describes his work *Rainbow 'Round My Shoulder* as "based on chain gangs dreaming of freedom symbolized in the shape of a woman." *Heartbeats*, a recent work for the José Limón Dance Company, utilizes international song and dance to illuminate the human connections. He continues to choreograph for major companies including as artistic mentor for the José Limón Dance Company and creating new works and resetting others for the Alvin Ailey and Cleo Parker Robinson companies.

Gus Solomons (1940–) and Garth Fagan (1940–) are two other outstanding black choreographers. Solomons, who danced in the Merce Cunningham Company before starting his own company, is known for his use of architectural form in his choreography. Fagan uses a combination of strong modern-dance technique, the distinct qualities of African movement, and black culture to choreograph dances. Garth Fagan Dance Company was formed in 1970. These significant artists all bring their experience as blacks to their unique choreographic statements. Donald Byrd (1949–) formed Donald Byrd/The Group in 1978 and now heads Spectrum Dance Theater, created in 1980 by Dale Merrill and based in Seattle. Byrd uses extreme physicality to express themes of gender, isolation, and culture.

Companies of Significant Influence in the 1960s and 1970s Paul Taylor (1930–) has also taken modern dance to new artistic levels. Taylor danced with Graham and Cunningham but has developed a style that is definitely his own. He is known for his choreographic wit, logical placings of movements, groupings of dancers, and satire. He has also created pieces that cleverly repeat a limited number of movements over and over again in unusual ways. He has not performed since 1974, but he still choreographs for his company extensively.

Bella Lewitzky (1916–) is unique to the world of modern dance because she made her international reputation as an artist in California instead of New York. Not since Denishawn had a modern-dance choreographer of major importance become established elsewhere than New York. Like Alvin Ailey, she was trained in California by Lester Horton. Her choreography is known for its powerful images and for extensive use of space, isolations, and quick movements. Lewitzky is always known for her extraordinary ability as a performing artist.

During the 1960s, modern dance reflected the social and political unrest that pervaded the decade. Many changes occurred. The only consistent characteristic was a discarding of the idea of theatricality for the use of everyday, pedestrian movement. Some dancers and choreographers were saying no to the idea of modern dance as it then existed.

Many times, traditional leotards, tights, and theatrical costumes were discarded and replaced by utilitarian garments such as overalls and hard hats, gym shorts and tennis shoes, sweat shirts and jeans — or even nudity. The 1960s and 1970s produced new names for modern dance, including antidance, nondance, minimal dance, environmental dance, dance without walls, verbal dance, and alternate space dance. Dance was sometimes performed in nontraditional spaces such as museums, malls, parking lots, parks, streets, and country clubs. Such spaces change the way dance is performed, and many times the dance is directed and choreographed by a dancer but performed by dancers and nondancers alike.

These periods of fertile creativity were characterized by a fresh look at time, space, and sound. Much of the movement was not on the proscenium stage (the *proscenium* is the floor separating the dancers from the audience and includes the arch and curtain). In this form, ordinary movement by ordinary people in ordinary places is considered valid as art. Many dancers collaborated on an equal basis with composers and studio artists to create pieces, or "events," as they were sometimes called. Before this generation of dancers, choreographers gave ideas to a composer or designer and then waited for the results. Now the collaboration often took place simultaneously, with all the artists contributing to the work.

As the decade of the 1970s drew to a close, two distinct camps of modern dance existed. One camp became more and more technically oriented and produced dances that were more and more difficult to perform. Dancers needed to study for periods of time with a choreographer in order to develop the style and technique needed to perform that choreographer's works. These choreographers followed more directly the established artists of the generation who had preceded them. They did not necessarily create in the same way that their teachers had, but they used many of the preceding generation's methods and ideas to create their own original works. Some of the artists involved with the more theatrically motivated modern dance of the 1970s were Murray Louis, Jennifer Mueller, Bill Evans, Cliff Keuter, Twyla Tharp, Lar Lubovitch, Gloria Newman, and Pilobolus.

The other camp became more and more antidance. Time, space, and energy were altered to make new forms, meanings, and nonmeanings in the modern dance. Most of these choreographers had also studied and worked with the preceding generation of choreographers, but they discarded many of that generation's ideas to do new, different, exciting things in dance. A few of the artists involved with this camp of modern dance in the 1970s were Don Redlich, Rudy Perez, Meredith Monk, Kei Takei, and Anna Halprin.

The Judson Group and the Grand Union Group were instrumental in expanding modern dance performance to include many of these new ideas. Both these groups pushed the boundaries of modern dance and influenced new artists to expand their notions of what dance could be. The Judson Group was a coalition of choreographers, dancers, and other artists who worked and performed from 1962 to 1968 in the Judson Church in New York City. This collective was composed of a diversity of artists who interacted and created new ideas about a new kind of modern dance. The Judson was followed by the Grand Union from 1970 to 1976. Several of the artists belonged to both groups. Some ideas produced were the inclusion of improvisation within the performance of a dance piece; "marking" or walking through rehearsal and presenting this concept as legitimate performance; ever-developing dance pieces that would change with each performance; and the alteration of the order of sections of completed dance works each time they were performed. These and other concepts were important in the expansion of the concepts of modern dance. Some of the most important contributors to these movements were Yvonne Rainer, Steve Paxton, Douglas Dunn, and David Gordon.

In California, Anna Halprin (1920–) has been redefining modern dance since the late 1950s. Her contribution to the ever-changing and evolving nature of modern dance has influenced many dancers and artists.

Her work in AIDS and with cancer patients is an extension and evolution of her earlier work in improvisation and process. This work has set her apart as one of the major innovators in modern dance.

Trends in the 1980s   Modern dance in the 1980s was characterized by several trends. Dance technique became more difficult and specific. Some movements that might typically be associated with sports or nondance activities were incorporated into choreographed pieces and used as dance movement. One choreographer who might be defined in this way is Trisha Brown (1936–), who uses movements that seem to defy gravity. Pilobolus combines athleticism, traditional modern dance, and the support of another dancer's weight in unusual ways to produce often humorous dances. Dancers seem to defy gravity. This group creates choreography by group decision.

Another development in the eighties was the alteration of the proscenium theater stage with all types of materials, including water, peat moss, rocks, or leaves, on the stage floor. Pina Bausch (1940–) uses these materials to enhance and influence her intense, dramatic concept of modern dance. Japanese choreographer Kei Takei (ca. 1948–) uses such objects to intensify and project her concept of dance. One of her projects, entitled *Light,* is continually developing and evolving.

Another trend that became significant in the 1980s involves choreographers who consult with other artists in related fields to collaborate and produce works. Some of the more prominent choreographers who work in this manner are Martha Clarke, David Gordon, Lucinda Childs, and Molissa Fenley. These choreographers collaborate with set, costume, and lighting designers, music composers, video artists, and others. All of these artists work together to produce works that are based on movement but that also incorporate ideas from theater, art, and music. Several artists are responsible for the final product, with the choreographer usually conceiving and directing the entire production. This method differs from the traditional methods of production, in which designers are often not consulted until after the choreographer has conceived and developed the work alone.

Some choreographers compose their own music as well as their own dances and are known as a choreographer/composer. One such artist, Laura Dean (1945–), has made significant contributions to modern dance through her use of spinning and repeated strong rhythmical patterns. Another choreographer/composer is Meredith Monk (ca. 1942–), who uses her own musical compositions and has recorded CDs that have earned recognition by the musical establishment.

IMPORTANT COMPANIES

Many contemporary choreographers continually produce significant works and tour the United States and other parts of the world. The scope of this book allows for a brief discussion of only a few of these artists.

Mark Morris (1956–) has been lauded as one of the most influential choreographers for the future of modern dance. He has been critically acclaimed for his use of music, his understanding of many and varied dance forms, and his ability to create energetic, explosive, and sometimes outrageous dances. He uses all sizes and shapes of male and female dancers and does not necessarily use them in the traditional male/female roles. He may even reverse their roles on stage. He maintains his own modern-dance company, as well as choreographs extensively for opera and ballet companies.

Lar Lubovitch (1945–) uses movement that is defined for the human body. He considers his dancers to be more important to him than any other element in his choreography, so his dances are designed to be humanistic. The Bill T. Jones and Arnie Zane Company uses movement that often evokes startling images of playful violence, outrage, and sometimes warm, emotional gestures. Since the death of Zane in 1988, Jones (1952–) has become a seminal influence in modern dance. One of his major works, *Still/Here*, deals with the issues of AIDS, death, and living.

Trends in the 1990s   Modern dance continued to evolve and change in the nineties because of many influences, including decreased funding from governmental agencies for arts in the United States, less appeal to dance audiences and theater patrons, an influx of major and innovative foreign dance companies, and the devastating effect of the disease AIDS on the field.

Some choreographers—for example, Twyla Tharp (1942–)—have reestablished their own modern-dance companies after making innovative choreographic contributions to major ballet companies. Trisha Brown's company now performs in prestigious proscenium theaters to music by established composers. In the seventies, Brown created mostly without music and in alternative spaces.

Many international modern-dance companies regularly tour the United States, including Pina Bausch's Tanztheater Wuppertal from Germany, Netherlands Dance Theater from Holland, France's Maguy Marin and the Lyons Opéra Ballet, and the Butoh-based Sankai Juku from Japan. Other companies include Cloud Gate from Asia and LaLaLa Human Steps from Canada. These companies offer diverse views of modern dance, and all use extraordinary visual and theatrical effects with distinctive cultural viewpoints.

Several other themes dominated modern dance in the 1990s, including the use of throwing and catching the body with gymnastic and wrestling techniques as the basis for choreographic statement. Some productions included elements from tap dancing, rhythmical percussion, and folk forms to appeal to new audiences. The shows *Stomp* and *Riverdance* are examples of how modern dance continues to redefine itself by fusing other forms of movement with current practices to find contemporary modes of expression.

The vitality of developing modern dance is less dependent on the New York scene than in the past. In major cities, a number of dancers, choreographers, and small companies have established a new kind of dance based on the experience inherent to their locale. As these companies establish themselves, they tour to the dance capital, New York City, and internationally, bringing with them a new point of view on modern dance expression.

NEW MILLENNIUM

As dancers and choreographers explore new ways of moving and create more meaningful ways to communicate with the audience, modern dance changes, incorporates, and adopts these new ideas. The difference between the pioneers and the dancers of today is that today's dancers have a strong, proven foundation from which to work.

Modern dance of the twenty-first century has continued in the tradition of the pioneers of the movement. Many successful companies in the twenty-first century have pushed the boundaries of former aesthetic guidelines and sensibilities. An example of this kind of stretching of aesthetic boundaries is Elizabeth Streb (1950–), who bills herself as an action architect/choreographer. Her work is based on extreme acrobatics, often with mats, horizontal bars, springboards, trampolines, and other circus equipment. The terms "Action Mechanics" and "Action Mavericks" are used to describe her dancers. Some of the names of the pieces performed by the company are *Squirm, Against the Wall,* and *Fly,* which aptly describe the movement in the dances. Some of the older established companies still performing on a regular basis include the companies of José Limón, formed in 1945; Paul Taylor, founded in 1954; and Mark Morris, founded in 1980.

Other modern dance companies regularly performing in this century include Hubbard Street Dance Chicago, founded in 1977 by Lou Conte (1942–); Momix, by Moses Pendleton (1949–), founded in 1981; Pilobolus, created by Alison Chase with Moses Pendleton in 1971 (cofounder Jonathan Wolken); the David Parsons Dance Company, created by David Parsons (ca. 1955–) in 1987; the White Oak Dance Project, founded by Mark Morris and Mikhail Baryshnikov (1950–) in 1990; Twyla Tharp Dance (1967–); and Lar Lubovitch Dance Company, formed in 1968.

Modern dance continues to change, evolve, and reflect the time in which it is created. It is influenced by societal issues, political concerns, the history of the art form, evolutions in the other arts, and the expansion and development of dance technique. Modern dance continually grows, develops, and reflects the moment of its creation and creator. This is the amazement and excitement of the art form.

GLOSSARY

eurythmics   pg. 67

expressionism   pg. 64

Labanotation   pg. 67

Chapter 6
Improvisation

The Process is the Purpose . . . Nonseparation
of life and art.

ANNA HALPRIN

Bill T. Jones/Arnie Zane Dance Company, Still/Here. *Photo © 1997 Johan Elbers.*

Creativity is important to problem solving in many disciplines, including science, business, the arts, and other areas. Creative solutions to problems significantly enrich our society and our institutions. The nurturing of the **creative process** is an essential part of dancers' education and an essential part of empowering their creative resources. Improvisation and choreography are two structured methods for fostering creative potential that individuals can use in their approach to dance and movement.

Given the revolutionary nature of its history, modern dance is in a strong position to be one of the best dance techniques for developing creativity in dancers. Dance has been described as an art form in which a dancer moves through space and time with dynamic and expressive movement qualities. Your body structure and movement potential, your senses and emotions, and your life experiences, attitudes, and intentions all contribute to the way you move both in your daily life and in your dance movements. In short, it is the totality of your personal life movement experiences, including family, cultural, and historical influences, coupled with your own life experiences that comprise your potential **movement vocabulary**—that is, the resources you have to draw on for creative expression. In addition, specialized training in, for example, dance techniques, sports, weight training, gymnastics, social dance, world dances, yoga, and Pilates, contributes to your creative possibilities and increases your ability to sustain your improvisation over many years in numerous contexts. There are various movement exercises that you can do to develop your awareness of your postural body shapes, the interrelationships and connections of the body parts, your relationship to space, and how your energy and intentions affect movement qualities and expression.

FINDING NEW WAYS TO MOVE

Where does movement originate? An important primary source is yourself. Movement experienced with no expectation of right or wrong results can be an effective method to begin the development of your own movement style and to begin to know how you want to express your inner feelings through movement. It is important that you develop awareness of yourself and commit to the discovery of the uniqueness of your own body structure in order to find how your body structure enables you to move most effectively. It is also important to nurture your movement preferences and expressivity. If you involve yourself in the spirit of improvisation, eventually you will find the way of moving that "feels right" for your body, based on all you have experienced in life. Sensitive self-exploration fosters your own creative understanding. In addition, establishing a strong partnership with your teacher as your guide and mentor in conjunction with your own self-knowledge will increase your potential for achieving your dance goals and dreams.

Dance **improvisation** serves some of the same purposes for a dancer as those served by an artist who sketches the outline of a visual image, a musician who "jams" without a written score, or a group of actors who dialogue without a script. Each participant gains in spontaneity, unforeseen insights, enhanced skills in quick responses, intuition, and a better sense of the particular medium, whether it be art, music, drama, or dance. Dance improvisation aids you in finding new ways to move, develops your technical skills, and provides another means to develop as an artist.

Basically there are two kinds of improvisation: structured and nonstructured. In **nonstructured improvisation,** you simply move without an idea, plan, or theme. It is movement for the sake of movement. It is an opportunity to explore your movement preferences, to learn what movements work well with your body structure, and to experiment with changes in time, space, shape, and dynamic qualities. In this kind of improvisation, there is no right or wrong, no judgments of what others or even you might think of the movement. It is a way to begin the process of developing your own confidence and personal expressive "voice" by creating movement out of movement that feels right to you and right for your body. You can begin this kind of improvisation by standing in a room or studio and quietly, meditatively listening to where you are in your feelings and thoughts and in your body at this moment. When the urge to move happens, let the movements flow sequentially out of what feels natural to you. Don't force yourself to move in any predetermined way. This was the way the late modern-dance choreographer Doris Humphrey began her exploration, leading to the development of her fall-recovery technique.

In **structured improvisation,** you establish a movement idea that may be simple or complex, for example, simple changes in the timing of the movement or a more complex narrative story line of some kind. At first you can begin to develop the movement idea through free exploration. As the improvisation continues, you may want to make some deliberate choices about the movement to determine whether you are establishing your idea through movement. Later, if a phrase of movement feels particularly satisfying, you may want to try to repeat it in some way. As you develop your skills at improvisation, you may want to capture some of your movement phrases so that you can repeat them. Many choreographers start with free movement exploration until they find the right movements to express their choreography ideas. At that point they need to be able to repeat the phrases that came out of the choreographic exploration. You can begin this kind of improvisation by defining some simple idea you can express in movement. It may be something about space, such as reaching in space above, below, forward, backward, and sideward; or a mood state like excited; or maybe changes in sounds created with your body by clapping, stomping, tapping, or vocalization.

Improvisation can be done alone or with others. It may be a single partner or a large group. Whether working alone or with others, the goal is still to move with sensitivity to your own body and movement preferences within the guideline of the improvisation. Working with a group requires an awareness of your relationship to the others spatially, how they are moving, and when your senses suggest it is appropriate to lead the group dynamic or how you can sensitively contribute to the unfolding of the group's creative process. Group improvisations can provide an excellent insight into the group process and the collective creative development of an idea. It can be a tool for choreographers to develop a dance work. Choreographer Steve Paxton is credited with starting a new dance form in the mid-1970s called **Contact Improvisation,** which raised improvisation to a potential art form.

Paxton's Contact Improvisation utilized pedestrian movements and various influences, including child's play, martial arts, sports, and social context. The concept spread to any number of groups and participants in Europe and North America. Speaking very generally, it was concerned with contact with a partner or partners, contact with the floor with different parts of the body, taking and giving body weight to others, touching and balance with awareness of gravity, and finding the easiest pathways to mutually facilitate body interactions. The only rule was that contact could not be made with the hands, thereby increasing the need for sensitivity to the demand and response to spontaneous actions of other dancers' bodies and their movement signals and cues.

BODY AWARENESS PROCESS

Following are some preliminary experiential personal explorations that might aid you in preparing for working in an improvisational situation. They might give you some ideas in how you process movement. Movement process is your particular method of organization and the steps you go through to arrive at a movement *gestalt* — that moment when all things come together to increase your clarity. Also, they may make you more **body aware,** that is, sensitive to how your body functions and organizes itself, uses space, and shapes itself and your habitual patterns of energy dynamics. These kind of quiet, unrushed, self-reflective experiences may reinforce your **movement recall** abilities in learning movement, rehearsing movement, and enhancing your own improvisations and choreography.

1. Lie on the floor in a relaxed position. Be sensitive to your body.

2. Be aware of your breathing, inhaling and exhaling, and notice what is happening in your body as a result of the breathing cycle. Be aware of how the body is internally and externally shaping itself as a result of how you are breathing. Try breathing through the vertical, width, and breadth of the body separately and then breathing through all three dimensions simultaneously, so you feel the body expanding in the dimensions similar to the inflation and deflation of a balloon.

3. Take some time to think about and sense the weight of your body supported by the floor.

4. Without moving, think about each part of your body. Imagine how each part can move through space and how each part is related to the whole body. For example, your upper leg bone is inserted into the hip socket at the pelvis and can move in all directions with or without rotation. The upper leg bone is attached to the lower leg bone, which primarily bends in only one direction and is in turn attached at the ankle joint, which leads down into the various movable bones of the foot. Think about how the pelvis/hip and heel connection facilitates movement.

5. Think about the length of the spine and how it connects the trunk to the head and down through the upper back, lower back, and into the pelvis. Think about how the lower and upper spine connection facilitates movement.

6. With the legs extended, **flexing** and **extending** in the ankle joints, set the body into a rocking motion—and be aware of the heel, pelvis, head connections. Check your body to see if you are holding tensions anywhere.

7. With the knees up and bent, pulled toward the pelvis, rock the pelvis forward, backward, and sideward. The forward and backward motion is like the pathway created by a playground swing; the sideward motion is like the sideward rotation of a car's steering wheel. Do the sideward motion alternating with one hip up and one hip down, and be aware of how the body is affected by pelvic initiation.

8. Quietly lie on the floor and reflect on a significant past event; remember where you were and what you felt about the occasion. Let this reflective imagery lead your body to an awareness of how you felt then and feel now.

Improvisational Exercises   Following are some improvisational exercises that may supplement the work given in the classroom. Try to do them when you are alone. Allow yourself plenty of time with each part of an exercise so that you don't feel rushed. Don't feel that you have to accomplish something, because there are no right or wrong results. When you are doing improvisation, you are trying to find out as much about your body as possible while moving through space and time with energy and expression.

The first two exercises may help you get in touch with your own body, body weight, and body rhythm.

1. Start lying on the floor. Take some time to sense your body. Are there any tensions anywhere? Stretch your body from head to foot, open the arms and legs wide to the side, and then relax. Repeat several times. Try to get a sense of what is happening in the body as you stretch and relax. Next, be aware of the shape of your body and how each part relates to the other parts of your body. Move to new lying positions and again note the changing body shape and the relationship of the body parts.

Next, lying on your back, be aware of each part of your body in contact with the floor. Be aware of the weight of your body. Slowly lift and then lower various parts of your body, for example, an arm, a leg, and parts of the torso. Be aware of the weight of the body part and the kind of energy required to lift and lower it. Try the same kind of actions while lying on your back and your sides, and be aware of how the movement actions are changed.

Next, to sense your breath rhythms and how the body lengthens and widens in space, take a few moments to concentrate on how your body moves when you inhale and exhale. Without forcing, lengthen your body from the top of the head to the toes as you inhale, and shorten your body from the head to the toes as you exhale. Repeat this a number of times, and then vary the idea by widening your body as you inhale and narrowing your body as you exhale. Finally, imagine the inner space of the torso as a large bell. Vocalize the vowels, a, e, i, o, u, and try to sense the sound as an internal changing body shape that is filling up the inner volume of the body. Explore the sound as originating from the areas of the pelvis, abdomen, chest, neck, or head. Be aware of how the sound, your breath, and your body all mutually support one another.

Next, to get a sense of your own rhythm, gently roll each part of your body from side to side on the floor — the head, a leg, an arm, the torso, and so forth. Be aware of the sensation of the movement and your body in contact with the floor. Next, gently roll the whole body from side to side and eventually roll over like a log being rolled. Next, to get a sense of your body weight working with gravity, again be aware of your breathing. As you inhale, lift your head off the floor, and as you exhale, lower your head to the floor. Without straining as you inhale, lift the pelvis off the floor, and as you exhale, let the movement subside onto the floor. Repeat this action with the whole torso, being aware of the length of the spine. Continue this rising and lowering, rising higher with each inhalation until you come to a standing position.

2. Standing up, try to be free of any unnecessary tension in your body. Stand as still as possible and try to determine whether any subtle, involuntary motion is taking place in your body in response to the demands of standing upright. Try the same thing standing on both feet with eyes closed, standing on one foot, and standing on the balls of the feet. Next, again be aware of your breathing. Without forcing, lengthen your body upward as you inhale, and lower your body as you exhale. Next, as you inhale, rise to the balls of your feet and stretch your arms overhead; as you exhale, fall forward and catch your weight on one foot. Return to standing on both feet. Shift your pelvis forward in order to fall forward; again, shifting the pelvis in each direction, fall to each side and to the back. Repeat. Make certain the whole body is involved, and note the kind of energy you are using as you rise, fall, and recover. Repeat the action again with a rhythm of some kind—for example, rise, fall, recover, pause; rise, fall, recover, pause. Next, try varying the rhythm, for example, rise-rise-rise (slow), fall (fast), recover (fast), or rise (fast), fall-fall-fall (slow), recover (fast). The rate or speed of the movement may change its dynamics or quality. If so, try to sense how your body adapts to the changing dynamics.

3. This exercise may help you get a sense of the space around your body and how you can move through it. Stand quietly and visualize all the space around your body in front, in back, to the sides, above, and below. Imagine that the space has the consistency of the sculptor's modeling clay. From every direction, gather the space into yourself. Then mold or give shape to the imaginary clay—for example, various sizes of spheres, cubes, and so forth. Clearly indicate the size and weight of the molded object. Be aware of the rhythm of your actions as you knead, shape, pat, and smooth the "clay." Next, tear the molded space into small pellets and hurl them or scatter them individually in every direction around your body.

Next, try scattering or throwing imaginary objects, for example, a feather, a leaf, a marble, a shotput, a coin, or a piece of paper. Be aware of the kind of energy required to throw each object. Next, imagine how each object would move through space and settle to the ground. Imagining your body as the thrown object, try to move and settle the same way. Involve the whole body, and make the movements as broad as possible. This exercise should help you avoid making fragmented movements.

TABLE 6.1   Constructing a Movement Phrase

Time	Body shape	Movement direction	Floor pattern	Mood feeling
slow	spread out	over	figure eight	alert
prolonged	closed in	under	zigzag	fear
fast	knotted	through	branched out	calm
instantly	voluminous	retreat	meander	joyful
slow-fast	tall	advance	circle	suspicious
fast-slow	short	toward	spiral in	proud
timeless	curved	away	spiral out	bold
time limit	angular	rise (up)	wavelike	courageous
leisurely	pin	sink (down)	straight	flirtatious
rushed	ball	sideward	diagonal	triumphant
held back	growing	diagonals	square	grief
frozen	diminishing	around	triangle	angry

Image	Action	Action	Position in room	Mood feeling
melting	crouch	pull	center	agitated
floating	throw	press	front of center	sheepish
jerking	catch	strike	back of center	repulsed
bumping	crawl	slash	left of center	nervous
bubbling	drop	dab	left front	defiant
pulsating	swing	flick	left back	furtive
stirring	rock	spiral	right of center	terrified
scratching	turn	shake	right front	giddy
cutting	bounce	squeeze	right back	pompous
pounding	jump	wring	hanging	surly
caressing	stretch	glide	lying	brooding
restraining	twist	pounce	edges	impatient

4. This exercise can help you develop a movement phrase. Select one word from each list in Table 6.1 and write the ten words sequentially on paper. Without preplanning, move your whole body in the way the ten-word description suggests. Keep repeating the sequence until you have a phrase that feels natural to you and that seems to have a beginning, a middle, and an end.

Write down two more word sequences with one word selected from each of the ten columns. Develop two more movement phrases. When you have established three movement phrases, try to give each one a beginning, a conclusion, and a transition into the next sequence. Decide whether any of the movements could be enriched by being performed another way and whether some movements ought to be eliminated or repeated a number of times. "Editing" one's work is an important function of the choreographer. Movements must be discarded if they do not contribute to the whole phrase or theme.

5. Initiate a series of movements by isolating one part of the body and using that part as an impetus to set your body in motion. The body part propels you through space in some direction, and you follow through until the movement comes to a conclusion. For example, let the head thrust backward, forward, or sideward, and let the rest of the body follow after the head has initiated the motion. Try the same with the pelvis, whole torso, shoulders, arms, legs, and so forth. Try moving in all of the different directions around your body.

6. Playing a game of red light/green light, move about the room quickly on the imaginary green light and come abruptly to a stop on the imaginary red light. Vary the timing of the stops and starts, and be aware of how your body reacts to the time element.

7. Imagine yourself walking in a swimming pool with the water up to your neck; then imagine yourself as an astronaut walking through weightless space. Be aware of how one restricts and the other frees the flow of your movement.

8. Imagine yourself in a vat of grapes. Crush the grapes with your feet; then lightly step on the grapes in another vat so that you do not crush any of them. Be aware of how your pelvis and center of gravity are involved in your exploration of weight.

9. Choose a spot in the room, and with total focus and attention, go directly to that spot. Next, walk forward while reaching behind you with one arm and looking to the side at some spot in the room. Try to focus your attention on all three directions at the same time, setting up a spatial conflict between your desire and intention to go in all three directions at once. Ask yourself how this affects your attitude toward directness and indirectness in the space you are moving through.

Exercises Combining Emotions, Ideas, Images, and Atmosphere

Emotions, ideas, images and atmosphere can be used separately or together, or they can be combined with other approaches. Here are some examples of their use together:

1. Imagine yourself in a room full of strangers on a hot, humid day. Thread your way through the room without touching the people. Exaggerate the adjustments your body makes to avoid contact.

2. Imagine yourself in a brightly lit room. Suddenly the lights go out; you hear strange noises that you finally realize are being made by the walls closing in on you. The walls close in until they have forced you into a tiny ball on the floor. Express your reactions to these events with movements that are as exaggerated as you can make them.

3. Move your whole body broadly through some everyday actions, such as brushing your teeth, sewing, clipping your nails, brushing your hair, or twisting the cap off a bottle.

4. Crouch on the floor, making yourself as small as possible. Then slowly unfold your body and spread out in every direction until you fill the entire room. Now reverse the action. Repeat the sequence, with a sense of joy as you rise and a sense of grief as you descend. Repeat again, rising like a roaring brush fire and descending as if your body has turned to liquid.

5. Remember how you felt this morning when you got out of bed. Walking around the room, try to get the same feeling in your movements. Exaggerate the movements and sustain the mood as you walk freely around the room.

USING IMPROVISATION IN THE CLASSROOM

Solo, duet, and group improvisation might or might not be used by your teacher in some way in the classroom. Some teachers at some point in the training process introduce improvisation as another approach to developing your awareness of working with a partner or a group. In the mid-1970s, Contact Improvisation became a performance form in dance with similarities in movement to the improvisation of musicians with sound or actors with words.

Partner Awareness Exercises   Following are **partner awareness** exercises that can be tried out with a dance classmate. Take your time doing the exercises. Be aware of and sensitive to your partner's movements and to how, cooperatively, you can make the movement experience meaningful to each of you. Face your partner in each exercise.

The first set of exercises experiments with weight and the second with **leading-following.**

Weight

1. Face each other about three feet apart, feet comfortably balanced, arms forward and slightly bent with palms resting against your partner's palms. Take turns passively leaning forward into your partner's palms, allowing your partner to support your weight. Try to develop a trust in passively giving your body weight and receiving your partner's body weight.

2. Balance yourself with one leg forward and one leg backward. As above, with palms together, take turns actively pressing your weight against

your partner's palms. Try to develop a sense of the give and take of sharing the pressure of actively using your own body weight or actively yielding to the body weight of your partner.

3. With feet comfortably together and knees bent, hold hands at the wrist and lean back away from each other. Experiment with sensitivity using each other's weight to oppositionally shift the weight forward, backward, and sideward, eventually cooperatively moving downward, with control, to sit on the floor.

Leading and Following

1. Facing each other with only the fingertips touching, take turns slowly moving, with one partner doing a free pattern of movement and the other following. Explore the **three-dimensional** space in front of you upward, downward, and sideward. Explore different spatial patterns, both linear and circular.

2. Facing each other a comfortable distance apart, repeat exercise 1 above without being in contact. Think of your movements as being a mirror image of your partner's movements. As you move, be sensitive to allowing your partner to sense, anticipate, and follow your moves. Take your time and allow your partner to share in your movement qualities and choices.

Tips for Classroom Improvisation
If your teacher works with improvisation, he or she will have a particular way of conducting improvisations. Some teachers incorporate them into a technique class, while others include them in a separate composition class or some other format. In beginning improvisation, some dancers feel shy or embarrassed about moving freely in front of others in the class. This feeling can be overcome. The sooner it is overcome, the more pleasure and rewards will result from the experience.

When your teacher gives you directions for an improvisation, listen carefully. When you are ready to begin, do not plan your movements ahead of time. Let them flow naturally based on the instructions given. Try to stay within the structure outlined. Avoid trying to imitate some movement sequence you have seen or learned elsewhere. Try to let things happen naturally without forcing them to happen. Don't be concerned about how the movement looks to others who might be watching. Concentrate on what you are doing. Remember that this is your own movement experience and that later your teacher can give you helpful suggestions. The more you improvise, the easier it becomes.

Whether or not your teacher does improvisation does not matter; exploring some of the ideas suggested in this chapter can help you find a way of moving that is unique because it originates from you and you alone.

BENEFITS OF IMPROVISATION

Improvisation can be focused in many different ways to achieve different goals and to develop your dance appreciation and awareness. Improvisation has many benefits:

1. Immediate accumulation, analysis, and synthesis of information to make decisions about movement, space, time, groupings, and group interactions.
2. Discovery of new movement and a lessening of reliance on preconceived ideas about movement.
3. Development of your awareness as a performer.
4. Experience of various concepts of movement and dance.
5. Development of your creative responses within the performance structure.
6. Development and use of a movement vocabulary.
7. Refinement of sensory and rhythmical acuity.
8. Development of movement recall for choreography.
9. Exploration of the senses, emotions, and feeling states.
10. Increased knowledge and understanding of the body in space and time.
11. Development of receptiveness to others when working within a group.
12. Development of the ability to find creative solutions to challenges.
13. Introduction to the choreographic process and structure.
14. Self-development and discovering your movement gifts.
15. Development of your own creative voice.
16. Expansion of personal creative potentials.
17. Exploration of movement patterns and themes.
18. Recognition of habitual movement patterns.
19. Development of enhanced coordination and poise.

Not only will improvisation enrich your dance experience, but it will also carry over into other areas of your life and help you develop an ability to use creativity in problem solving.

GLOSSARY

Chapter 7
Choreographic Approaches

Each dance is unique and free, a separate organism
whose form is self-determined.

MARY WIGMAN

Mark Morris Dance Group, Dido and Aeneas. *Photo by D. Pierre.*

Some students ask, "Why should I study choreography when all I want to do is dance?" It's true that a brilliant dancer may never have choreographed anything, and a brilliant choreographer may have been a poor dancer. A successful performer, however, doesn't just dance. You dance about something or to express something, even when the dance is without a plot. If you hope to make a statement with your body that reflects your intentions or those of the choreographer, you should have some idea of the choreographic structure behind the dance you are doing. If you want to teach dancing or to choreograph someday, you can save yourself countless hours of aimless experimentation by knowing a few techniques for how to begin your experiments.

Improvisation and basic choreographic forms might be as much a part of your training as daily technique classes. Technique classes train the body. Improvisation frees your movement from the restrictions placed on it by a codified technique and frees your own creative energies. Knowledge of choreographic structures trains your mind and sharpens your critical faculties and perceptions.

What are the basic things you will have to do if you choreograph? It helps to keep an open mind to ideas, awareness of your world, and sensitivity to yourself. Your viewpoint and perspective will define your choreography as, perhaps, quirky, profound, satirical, entertaining, or something else unique. One essential thing is to be yourself and find your artistic voice; your teacher is an important guide to your goals.

Along the way you will need to *explore* movement, *select* and *decide* on the movement you want to use, and then put it in a *coherent order* to share with your audience. You will have to make decisions on whether or not your idea will be better as a solo, duet, trio, or group work and whether or not you want to start choreographing for yourself or others. A solo work requires a different kind of emphasis than a group work, which you need to consider. Most of all, explore and find your voice.

There are many ways to choreograph. You will find the way that works best for you. We present here only a few basic approaches to choreographic exploration.

DESIGN

A sense of body design in space and good stage balance comes with experience. You can do a number of things to develop your "artistic eye" for line, form, shape, and theatrical drama.

Observing Design   Pictures are telegraphic. They tell you a story without the addition of a caption below them. Dance should be able to do the same. Try the following exercises to help develop your artistic eye:

1. Look at paintings of different periods of history. Observe how the artist has placed the people in relationship to one another, how the people are posed, and why their clothes make them stand out the way they do.

2. Study the pictures in pictorial magazines such as *National Geographic* or *Smithsonian* and see why some pictures and advertisements hold your attention.

3. Look at the pictures of athletes in "frozen" motion and trace the natural lines of their movement.

4. Look at the buildings or the landscape around you and ask what is beautiful, interesting, or jarring about it.

If you want to dance about people and their universal concerns, you have to understand them and what makes them behave as they do in a given set of circumstances. The following exercises are a study of people and nature:

1. Watch how people of different ages and social classes walk, sit, and stand.

2. Observe how people move when they are happy, sad, or expressing some other emotion.

3. Watch how people in a social situation group themselves into a circle or how some sit off by themselves.

4. Watch how children, animals, and birds move and consider why they move that way.

5. Study the shapes formed by a tree, a leaf, a rock, or oil stains on a mud puddle.

6. Become acutely aware of your own senses. How do different textures feel? Be aware of odors, notice the taste of your food, really study how something looks (its shapes, its colors), and start to listen carefully to the sounds of nature and to human-made sounds.

7. Begin to notice natural movements, such as the sway of trees, the ebb and flow of waves, and the ripples in a pond. Try to sense the dynamics of the motion and how your body could suggest that movement and its dynamics.

All of life, all of nature, is potentially the concern of the artist, who must bring some kind of order out of the myriad possibilities through selection and emphasis. Basically, choreography can be thought of as planning movement of the human body through space and time. It requires choices in body movement and spatial design, rate of speed, rhythm, dynamics, and overall form. To have merit, the materials of dance need to be manipulated imaginatively rather than as a series of movements strung together without coherence. Developing appropriate movements takes time and discipline.

Choreographers work in many different ways, some letting the dance shape itself, others having clearly established ideas they wish to communicate. For the beginning choreographer, it is usually helpful to define the theme of your study or work. It is helpful to consider what the content of the study will be, how it will develop logically, and what it will communicate. All sections should flow naturally into one another and should have coherence to the whole.

Kinds of Design   There are two basic modes of stage design: **symmetrical** and **asymmetrical.** In symmetrical design, the stage is equally balanced on both sides. For example, if you have two dancers on one side of the stage, then you have two dancers on the other side. In asymmetrical design, the stage is not balanced. If you have two dancers on one side of the stage, you might have four on the other side in staggered positions. Symmetrical design is the most pleasing to look at, but it becomes the dullest to look at if overused. Another kind of design is *dynamic design,* achieved by linear spacing of dancers or massed grouping; the first establishes the line; the second, a sense of volume or mass.

Dynamic design

Presumably you are choreographing for members of an audience, so you want to keep their eyes constantly "entertained" with unexpected movements, lines, shapes, and forms. There is nothing worse than putting your audience to sleep. There are no bad audiences—only bad dancers and bad choreographers. You have a responsibility to communicate something to a paying audience, even if it is outraged at what you have done. The worst thing you can do to your audience is cause indifference or boredom, unless that is your intention.

MOTIVE AND CHARACTER

Another approach to finding new movement or to defining a character in a dance work is to improvise by working from human stereotypes, from the psychological makeup of a specific person, or from gestures or common movement activities such as throwing a ball or by using an animal as a reference point for character definition.

If you are going to choreograph a part — a swaggering braggart, for example — you could ask yourself questions such as what motivates this person, what does he want, and how does he move. An easy way to begin is to decide that he acts like some animal, maybe a strutting rooster. You could then improvise around the idea of a rooster strutting with his chest pushed forward and his head quickly surveying all of his domain.

Gesture/Posture   A different approach to defining a braggart's character with movement is to improvise on some imaginary situation he might be in. For example, if he were in a room full of people and was offered food, how would he take the food from a tray and how would he eat it? Would he use small, delicate hand **gestures,** or would he totally surround the food with his whole body?

If the movement is to be repeated and set into dance for the character, it is helpful to decide first on a few extreme examples of how this person moves or exaggerated **postures** that he might assume, and then combine them, moving from one extreme posture to another or from movement pattern to movement pattern. You can eventually arrive at specific movements that get your idea across. The tendency with novice choreographers is to put everything they know indiscriminately into the dance. An audience will probably see the choreography only once and so must be carefully led to see the idea that you want it to see.

Abstraction of Character   You will not always choreograph or dance as a literal, recognizable character; sometimes you will dance or choreograph as an **abstraction** of an idea or character. The same methods of choreographic improvisation and definition described above can be utilized until you have arrived at the essence of what you want to say in movement. For example, if you pick a flower from a garden, you could go through the actual motions of picking a flower (literal gesture), or a stylized motion of picking a flower (pantomime), or an extended motion suggesting the picking of a flower, indicating the joy or nostalgia you feel rather than the actual picking of the flower (dance).

Emotion or Feeling   Sometimes it is useful to develop a movement **motif** that originates from your feelings. An example of a process working with feeling is to find and listen to a recording of a piece of music that evokes strong feelings or elicits some kind of imagery for you. Get in a comfortable position and listen to your selected music. Using crayons or colored felt pens, without preplanning, freely make patterns on a large blank piece of paper that are expressive of your feelings and your response to the music. Next, using some flexible colored wire, create a three-dimensional sculpture of the pattern you drew on the paper. When you have created the sculpture, move through the pattern from one end to the other. Do this until you have a repeatable movement pattern. As you are doing the movement pattern, try to bring your initial feelings into the movement.

Object   Sometimes it is useful to use an object that, for you, has a beautiful pattern — for example, a seashell, a dried branch from a tree, a crystal, or a sculpture. Trace your finger over the pattern many times until you have discovered the details of the pattern. See if you can find what the object symbolizes as a theme for you. By moving through the pattern while expressing your symbolic theme, you can establish a movement motif that has meaning for you.

Action Picture   From newspapers or magazines, find four or five still photographs of dancers or athletes caught in the frozen moment of an exciting action sequence. Attach the still photos to a blank paper in a sequence that you find interesting. Organically move from one static pose to the next, developing a spatial movement pattern that has a natural ebb and flow. Experiment with the change between poses in order to develop an exciting movement pattern. In performing your pattern, try to capture the spirit of what you originally found appealing in the **spatial tensions** and designs suggested in the photos.

FORMS

Many people have ideas but lack the ability to share them with others. You as a choreographer or dancer must develop the craft of organizing your ideas into some structure that will communicate them to the audience.

There is no easy formula that will guarantee success, but a few forms around which you can organize your ideas are presented here as possible starting points. (Some of these basic forms require more than one dancer.)

Motif   The motif (motive) is a brief, recognizable movement phrase or idea. Establishing for yourself clear movement motifs is useful before working with more complex forms listed below. You can start with an improvised movement phrase, repeating it many times, exaggerating various elements of the phrase, exploring changes in the texture of the phrase — percussive, sustained, smooth, crescendo-decrescendo, use of your space and body shapes — and finally editing the phrase until it represents the gist or quintessential expression of your idea, mood, or movement statement.

You can share it with a fellow student to find out if she or he sees the motif you are showing.

Theme   The **theme** is one of the most elemental forms. It is particularly useful when you begin to choreograph extended pieces. A theme makes some basic statement and is organized around some central movement idea. For example, using the idea of a "work theme," you could choreograph a movement pattern of eight bars, suggesting the movements of a lumberman chopping down a tree. The movement theme: He chops the tree.

Theme and Variation   The basic movement theme is shown once and then repeated with some kind of basic change. Common ways of doing the **variation** are

1. Slowing down the entire movement pattern.
2. Speeding up the entire movement pattern.
3. Inverting the movement (for example, movements that go up now go down, movements that came toward the body now go away from the body).
4. Reversing the movement pattern (that is, starting at the end and work-ing toward the beginning). *Retrograde* is the term used in choreog-raphy for this concept.
5. Extending the amount of time selected movements are performed.
6. Diminishing the amount of time selected movements are performed.
7. Embellishing or adding movement to the basic theme.
8. Eliminating movement from the basic theme.

Starting with the basic chopping theme and then doing each of these eight variations for eight bars, you would end up with a choreographic piece seventy-two bars long. In embellishing the basic theme, you might add the idea that the lumberman stops to wipe his brow with a handker-chief because of the heat or stops to sharpen the cutting blade or to watch the tree fall. By combining the basic theme with variations or with some other form, you can tell a story or suggest a change of mood or anything that you want to communicate, yet beneath it all is a basic structure that has a unity with your basic premise, the original eight bars of movement.

ABA   Another common form is ABA—the statement of a basic theme (A), a second theme (B), and a repetition of the original theme (A). The lumberman is chopping briskly with a steady rhythm in the first theme; in the second theme, he tires, and the chopping slows down and changes rhythm frequently; then he gets a "second wind" and again chops briskly with a steady rhythm.

Fugue   The fugue requires two or more dancers. In the beginning, each dancer shares a single theme and moves in imitation of the beginning of that theme. As the movement progresses, ultimately the two or more dancers' themes develop independently of one another to establish their own movement identity. For example, all dancers might do the eight bars of chopping and then develop the chopping theme in his or her own way to establish an independent movement sequence.

Sonata   The sonata form is made up of two themes, primary and secondary, plus a recapitulation or joining of the two themes. For example, in theme 1, the man chops the tree. In theme 2, the man watches the tree fall. In the recapitulation, the man again chops the tree and watches it fall. In such a recapitulation of the two themes, you might have the idea of felling a forest and not merely one tree.

Round   The round is a common form exemplified by the song "Three Blind Mice." Each dancer is of the same physical or emotional type. The same theme is repeated a number of times, with new dancers joining in at some point. The beginning dancer finishes first; then the other dancers stop as they finish the same movement pattern. For example, the man chops the tree (movement A), the man wipes his brow (movement B), and the man watches the tree fall (movement C). In a simple round, the first dancer starts at movement A, continues through movements B and C, and stops. The second dancer begins at movement A when the first dancer begins movement B and continues to the end and stops. The third dancer begins movement A when the second dancer begins at movement B and continues to the end and stops. The first dancer, instead of stopping at the end of movement C, may introduce new movement themes that are repeated by the second and third dancers.

Canon   The canon form is similar to the round except that all the dancers finally join in the same movement to bring it to an end (coda). The movement is done by two or more dancers, each beginning slightly after the preceding one. The French song "Frere Jacques" is an example of a canon. In a dance canon, each new dancer does the movement exactly as the original movement was done, but the new dancer may be a different physical or emotional type from the original dancer. In the original theme, the lumberman chops the tree. In the successive repeats of the theme, he may be joined by his wife and then by his son.

Counterpoint In counterpoint, two independent themes are danced against one another. The lumberman chops the tree while someone builds a house using the material the lumberman has produced.

Chance Composition Choreography by chance is called a form here because the artist must still select and shape the final piece. One common example is placing a certain number of movement instructions written on individual pieces of paper into a box, then drawing them out one at a time and assembling them into a movement pattern in the same order they were drawn out. For example, you might draw out these instructions (1) move in a circle, (2) make percussive movements, and (3) exhale. Using the idea of the lumberman, you might have him circle the tree, chop it sharply, and exhale with fatigue. It should be understood, however, that choreography by chance usually implies the lack of a preconceived theme.

All of these forms could, of course, be built around some other theme — abstract, literal, or movement oriented.

TIME AND MUSIC

Time As a choreographer, you need to develop an awareness of your personal sense of time, that is, your own inner rhythm that motivates the time duration of your movements. Your creative organization of the timing of the movements can enrich your choreographic expression. In one sense, time can be thought of metaphorically as a stream of water connecting what has been, what is now, and what will be in the future. Time has been associated with the changing seasons and years and, more recently, with the ever-present clock. Time is an important element of dance. How you perceive and structure the time elements in your choreography will influence how you interpret your personal perspective and convey it to both your dancers and the audience.

Music Traditionally, dance is performed to music or to structured sound of some kind. You may use prerecorded music, work with musicians or a composer, or create your own music or organized sounds. Whatever method you choose, you will need to know some of the language of music and how it is organized. Musicians do not necessarily know the language of dance, but dancers need to know about music. Your knowledge and creative interpretation of music or organized sound will enhance your choreographic intentions. One way of learning more about this craft is to follow a musical score while listening to the prerecorded score.

Measure   Music is organized into bars (measures). In the examples that follow, we have listed the most common musical meters that you are likely to encounter in your beginning work. (Notice that the "and" counts have been omitted.) The symbol > indicates the strong beat. The symbol ‿ indicates the secondary or moderate beat, which means that it is accented more heavily than the other counts but not as heavily as the strong beat. The two numbers written as a fraction constitute the musical time signature. The upper number shows how many counts there are in a bar, and the lower number shows what kind of durational value gets one count. In 2/4 time, for example, there are two counts to a bar and a quarter note gets one count. In dance, the upper number is more important.

Rhythm   Try clapping the following rhythms, accenting the first count to get their rhythmical feeling.

$\frac{4}{4}$ 1̇ 2 3̆ 4 | 1̇ 2 3̆ 4 | 1̇ 2 3̆ 4

(three bars of four counts each)

$\frac{3}{4}$ 1̇ 2 3 | 1̇ 2 3 | 1̇ 2 3

$\frac{2}{4}$ 1̇ 2 | 1̇ 2 | 1̇ 2 |

$\frac{6}{8}$ 1̇ 2 3 4̆ 5 6 | 1̇ 2 3 4̆ 5 6 | 1̇ 2 3 4̆ 5 6

Notice that the 6/8 rhythm has been stressed heavily on the first count and less heavily on the fourth count. Often a 6/8 rhythm is played very quickly by the musician, so it is frequently more easily counted by the teacher as 1̇ 2 | 1̇ 2 or 1̇ and a 2̇ and a.

The example below shows how the counts would be written in musical notation.

The modern dancer often experiments with changes in the rhythmical form. You may change the number of counts in the basic musical bars to give variety. You might dance to a series of bars such as 1̇ 2 3 | 1̇ 2 3 4 | or 1̇ 2 | 1̇ 2 3 or some other combination of rhythms. This is referred to as **mixed meter.**

Another musical change you might use is called **shifted accent.** Instead of falling on the first count, the accent falls on another count. For example:

$$\overset{>}{1}\ 2\ 3 \mid \overset{>}{1}\ 2\ 3 \mid 1\ \overset{>}{2}\ 3 \mid 1\ 2\ \overset{>}{3}$$

$$1\ 2\ \overset{>}{3} \mid \overset{>}{1}\ \overset{>}{2}\ 3 \mid \overset{>}{1}\ 2\ 3 \mid \overset{>}{1}\ 2\ 3$$

Here the expected heavy accent in the third, fourth, fifth, and sixth bars has been shifted to a count other than the first count. This example shows a rhythmic concept called **syncopation** — a displacement of accents onto beats of the measure that are not usually emphasized.

Cumulative rhythm occurs when each succeeding bar has one more count added to it. For example: $\overset{>}{1} \mid \overset{>}{1}\ 2 \mid \overset{>}{1}\ 2\ 3 \mid \overset{>}{1}\ 2\ 3\ 4$. **Subtractive rhythm** is the exact opposite of cumulative rhythm. Each succeeding bar has one count subtracted from it. For example: $\overset{>}{1}\ 2\ 3\ 4 \mid \overset{>}{1}\ 2\ 3 \mid \overset{>}{1}\ 2 \mid \overset{>}{1}$.

Hemiola is a regular displacement of accent that temporarily produces a new time signature. For example: $^{6}_{8}\ \overset{>}{1}\ 2\ \overset{>}{3}\ 4\ \overset{>}{5}\ 6$.

Dancers do not always dance with the strong recurring beat of the music. This would soon lead to boredom. To add interest, the dancers also move on the "offbeat" or against the prevailing rhythm. If you clap the counts below with the accents indicated above them, you will feel the sense of **double time,** or doubling of the basic beat. Each bar should take exactly the same amount of time to clap:

$\overset{>}{1}\ 2\ \overset{>}{3}\ 4,\ \overset{>}{1}$ and 2 and $\overset{>}{3}$ and 4 and, $\overset{>}{1}\ 2\ \overset{>}{3}\ 4,\ \overset{>}{1}$ and 2 and $\overset{>}{3}$ and
4 and

Common groupings of counts (musical notes) in a measure used in dancing are groups of 2s (2/4 time, two quarter notes, with two strong beats, or 6/8 time, six eighth notes, with two strong beats, each with sub-beats of 3), 3s (3/4 time), or 4s (4/4 time). See the examples below (a small u indicates an unaccented beat):

$$^{2}_{4}\ \overset{>}{1}\ \overset{u}{2} \mid \overset{>}{1}\ \overset{u}{2}$$

$$^{3}_{4}\ \overset{>}{1}\ \overset{u}{2}\ \overset{u}{3} \mid \overset{>}{1}\ \overset{u}{2}\ \overset{u}{3}$$

$$^{4}_{4}\ \overset{>}{1}\ \overset{u}{2}\ \overset{>}{3}\ \overset{u}{4} \mid \overset{>}{1}\ \overset{u}{2}\ \overset{>}{3}\ \overset{u}{4}$$

$$^{6}_{8}\ \overset{>}{1}\ \text{and}\overset{u}{a}\ \overset{>}{2}\ \text{and}\overset{u}{a} \mid \overset{>}{1}\ \text{and}\overset{u}{a}\ \overset{>}{2}\ \text{and}\overset{u}{a}$$

Another common musical grouping used in modern dance is the *triplet* — three quick movements done to one count of music:

$^{3}_{4}$	dance count:	1 2 3	1 2 3	1 2 3
	music count:	1	2	3

Dancers sometimes prefer to group a series of musical measures together to go with a longer phrase of dance movement, for example, an eight-count phrase combining two measures of 4/4 time. Or, in a fast 3/4 time such as a waltz, dancers may count each measure of three counts as only one count:

$$\begin{array}{c} 3 \\ 4 \end{array} \quad \begin{array}{l} \text{dance count:} \\ \text{music count:} \end{array} \quad \frac{1}{1\ \ 2\ \ 3} \ \Big| \ \frac{2}{1\ \ 2\ \ 3} \ \Big| \ \frac{3}{1\ \ 2\ \ 3} \ \Big|$$

To get a feeling in your body of these musical concepts, connect the mixed-meter, shifted-accent, syncopation, and cumulative and subtractive rhythms into a movement phrase. Use broad, strong movements to illustrate each strong accent so that the structure of each bar is clear.

Tempo   Tempo refers to the speed of the musical accompaniment or dance movement. *Changes in tempo,* from very slow to very fast or the reverse, result in a change of the quality of the movement. Changes in tempo sometimes make otherwise dreary movement quite exciting to watch.

Common musical tempi, from very slow to very fast, are largo, lento, adagio, andante, moderato, allegro, vivace, presto. To keep track of where you are in the music and movement phrase, it might be helpful to number the measures as you are working, for example, measures 1234, 2234, 3234, 4234, and so forth.

MUSIC AND DANCE COMPOSITION

Music can add a great deal to your choreography, or it can destroy it. Following are a few things to keep in mind when you are working with music. (You might want to choreograph the dance in *opposition* to these ideas to achieve a dissonant look in your movement.)

1. Keep the qualities of the dance movement consistent with the mood of the music (or, for contrast, deliberately work against the mood of the music).

2. Analyze the structure of the music so that you can repeat the movements on the same counts or phrases twice running or so that you can teach the movement to someone else without being vague about what happens when. A pencil and paper are invaluable. Make dashes on the paper in accompaniment with the regular beats of the music until you have developed some kind of musical pattern to work from. As you listen over and over to the music, make notes above the dashes to indicate shifts in the rhythm, shifts in the mood, or the appearance of new instruments—or whatever other notes can guide you.

3. Try composing your own music. You might play it *while you are dancing* or have someone play it for you. You can use percussion instruments if they are available. If not, so much the better: find and use rocks, sticks, or dried leaves on a branch, or run a comb over paper. You can

discover exciting new sounds by trying out the least likely objects. Then organize the sounds into some repeatable form. If you have access to a tape recorder, you can record your music. A tape recorder makes it possible to use other sounds as well, for example, a ticking clock, an airplane, dripping water, or a cat's cry. Composing your own music frees you from the restrictions placed on you by the composer, and it can also be a lot of fun.

4. Find your own way of working with music that is best suited to your own creative needs. Ideally, dancers and choreographers need to know as much as possible not only about the wide range of types of music, both historical and contemporary, available to them, but also about what kinds of instruments produce what kinds of sounds. Radio, television, and recorded music are good sources for hearing music, from symphonic compositions to the latest musical innovations. Television is a good source for hearing and seeing which instrument is producing which sounds.

Anyone interested in choreographing should keep a journal to notate information about music that might be good for choreographing. In the same journal, you could jot down ideas or sketches of movement images you have. These jottings could be a useful resource at a later time.

THEATRICAL ELEMENTS: COSTUMES, PROPS, SCENERY, LIGHTING, AND SOUND

If you are going to wear a costume or use scenery and props, take advantage of them by analyzing their function in relation to your purposes. For example, if you are wearing a long cape, experiment to find out how many different ways you can move it or use it to augment the spatial designs of your body. Can it be used as a prop like a bullfighter's cape or placed on the floor to suggest a forbidden territory that no one dares to enter? The important thing to remember about a dance costume is that you don't just wear it but rather take advantage of its restrictions and use them to enhance your visual designs or enhance your ideas.

Costumes do not need to be expensive in order to be effective. Using your leotard and tights as a basic costume, you can perform wonders with pieces of unsewn material or dyes.

If you use stage props, explore all their possibilities. For example, an ordinary chair can be sat on, lain on, stood on, crawled under or over, or danced with like a silent partner. The list of uses is endless.

Costumes, props, and scenery make it possible to extend the potentials of your body design in space and to add new elements of stage interest. The only limitations to movement possibilities are those that come either from your not being imaginative or from your deliberately being selective.

Lighting for dance is very specialized and is an art unto itself. It is not the same as lighting a drama production. Ideally, you will be able to work with an experienced lighting designer who knows the requirements for dance. Two things to avoid are having the stage so dark that you can't clearly see the movements or, conversely, so bright that there is no shaping of the body. Lighting should reflect the mood of your work, enhance images, and focus attention on important movements.

Your choice of **sound** is crucial to the success of your work. If you use recorded music, the audio should be of the highest quality. If you work with live accompaniment, it is advisable to work with the musician/singer/musical ensemble to make sure their accompaniment is consistent so the dancers are not suddenly required to dance too fast or too slow compared to the tempo at which you rehearsed. You may want to experiment and create your own musical accompaniment, for example, by clapping, creating sounds vocally or on your own body, striking sticks or rocks together, or making your own musical instruments.

If you become discouraged in your experiments, keep in mind that even the most famous choreographers started at the beginning. No less than they, you have to work at your craft if you want eventually to use it to express your ideas and feelings.

FOCUS

As a choreographer, you need to establish for yourself and your audience the primary objective of the piece and how all the parts relate to the **basic focus** or purpose. In developing your dance movement, you and your dancers will need to find an **internal focus** and intention that motivates it. It is also important to clearly define for the dancers the **external focus** to the space and to the other dancers. As a choreographer, you need to develop your awareness of the spatial arrangement and the spatial movement of the dancers on the stage. They must know where, when, how, and why they enter or exit the performance space. Finally, you need to direct the **audience's focus** to what you want them to see at any given time.

Whether or not you intend to become a professional choreographer, you can gain knowledge about yourself and about the art of dance by developing organized movements into a piece that has meaning for you. Merce Cunningham once said that you should keep choreographing, and one day you will wake up to find that you have become a choreographer. Doris Humphrey stood quietly in the studio freeing herself of all she had learned and waited for the person in the mirror to reveal her own personal potential movement. Paul Taylor, as a student of art, brought his knowledge of art to his choreography. Alwin Nikolais brought his knowledge of music and technology to the development of a new way of organizing movement into a dance art. Choreographing is not like using a cookbook, turning to a page to find your recipe; it is a whole way of life.

You can learn the craft of choreography, but only you can bring your unique point of view to the creation of a dance work that is based on all you have experienced in your lifetime.

These are some ideas you can consider as you go through your choreographic process and as self-assessment for your process:

1. What is your choreographic goal, unifying theme, idea, or feeling of the dance?
2. What did you accomplish with the dance today, and how do you feel about it?
3. What did you like/dislike about your movements and why?
4. What do you think you could add, subtract, or change to make it better?
5. What movement phrases do you like, and how do they relate to your theme?
6. What did you do to assure a variety of movement choices in your choreography?
7. What are your choreographic ideas, and how do you solve them?
8. What did you learn about creating a dance?
9. What did you find challenging? How did you solve those challenges?
10. What connections does this have to your other classes?

In addition, it might be useful to ask yourself:

- What is this dance about — that is, what is its intended or perceived theme and focus?
- Is it better expressed as abstract, narrative, movement for movement's sake, entertainment, or something else?
- Is this a dance for you to explore or expand your own creative options, to creatively complete an assignment, to engage an audience, or something else?
- How can this work be enhanced through sound, lighting, costuming, props, or sets, whether in the studio, outdoors, or on the stage?
- With or without a budget, how can you manipulate the space and elements to achieve effects that further your theme?
- If you are working with dancers, are you providing them with an opportunity to share your process and to grow in their own process?

GLOSSARY

Chapter 8
Evaluation and Criticism

We have to meet the artist halfway. We have to bring
something before we can bring something away.

CLIVE BARNES

Donald McKayle Dance Company, Rainbow 'Round My Shoulder.

BEGINNING THE CRITIQUE

Often you hear people say of something they have seen, "I liked it" or "I didn't like it." This is the beginning of criticism. Unfortunately, most people never go beyond these statements to analyze *why* they liked or didn't like what they saw.

If you want to dance, choreograph, teach, or simply be an intelligent member of the audience, it is important to know why you liked or didn't like something and to be able to express your viewpoint intelligently. You can learn a great deal about what to do and what not to do in the dance theater by seeing dance concerts and by giving a critical **evaluation** of what you have seen. Your criticisms should never be exclusively negative or positive. You should impartially evaluate both the good and the bad features.

You may not be able to see dance concerts regularly, but you can increase your critical faculties and perceptions in other ways. Every movie, television show, advertisement, short story, and so on has a structure and makes a statement in some way, good or bad. You can apply the same principles to these communication forms that you do to dance. Each time you see a dance work, you are increasing your ability to judge and critique a dance.

Dance Description   As a student developing your critical skills, you can gain a clearer understanding of a dance work by a careful and responsible written description of the dance work, which generally will lead you toward a more confident assessment and judgment of the particular work you are critiquing. You can start by assessing from your own point of view what the most important effect or intention of the performance was. Did it evoke an emotional response from you or the audience? Works that are considered "great" touch us on some visceral level that we identify with and connect with on a common psychological or emotional level. Describe in detail what you saw, what you felt, and what you thought were the most important aspects and intention of the performance. Give specific examples and explain how they contributed to what you perceive as the choreographer's intention for the work. The beginning of critical analysis is to look at the work from your perspective and next to articulate your perspective in a written context. Analysis of others' works will enable you to be more self-aware and help you to critically examine your own work in a positive and informed way.

CRITERIA FOR EVALUATION

You can analyze the overall structure by asking yourself how it began, how it ended, and what happened in between. A well-structured **dance** should have a beginning, a development of the beginning, and a resolution. The

form may or may not be used to tell a story. Nevertheless, it should start somewhere, accomplish something, and be resolved.

With a professional company, you have the right to ask if the work was performed well and if the dancers contributed to the choreographer's conception. Many good works are ruined by bad dancers, and many bad works are effective when performed by good dancers. Was it theatrically exciting? There is no law that says art cannot be entertaining. The audience has a right to expect something more for its time and money than a pedestrian presentation.

Creative choreographers make a personal, unique dance statement that sets their dance work apart from other choreographers' works. In viewing a dance, you might be able to categorize it in a general way that will help you gain insights into the choreographer's perceptions about movement and how he or she has unified them into a cohesive whole. Does the work have a narrative story line, or is it abstract, with little or no attempt at pictorial representation? Do spectacle and technical display seem more important than the inventiveness of the dance movements? How have the choreographer and scenic and lighting designers established a mood, a locale, and an environment for bringing the viewer into the choreographer's vision? Has the choreographer used the music, sound, words, or silence in a way that reinforces both the audio and the visual aspects of the work?

Modern dance may be performed in many different kinds of **performance spaces.** The kinds of spaces used will influence the final shape of the dance. In developing your awareness and critical skills, it is helpful to analyze the performance space, how the choreographer has utilized the restrictions and potentials of that space, and whether or not the space has been transformed into an arena for theater-dance "magic" or something else.

Choreographers usually have a characteristic **style** achieved by the kind of movement choices they have made. Is the movement generally free, lyrical, and harmonious; is it restricted, angular, and disharmonious; or is it something else? How do the dancers move through the space, enter and exit, and organize themselves to the space or to the other dancers? How has the choreographer organized the duration of time and rhythm in the piece? What kind of emotions, moods, thoughts, or ideas do the dancers seem to be expressing, and are they expressing them through gestures, postures, or relationships among dancers, or in some other manner? How has the choreographer organized each section of the work, and how does each section relate to the whole?

The questions in the following lists can help you increase your critical and evaluative skills and give you ideas to consider when doing your own choreography.

The Dance as a Whole

1. Was there a unifying theme or concept in the dance that could be iden-tified? If so, what was it? If not, how could the choreographer have made it clearer?

2. Did the concept of the work have relevance for you? Why do you think the theme was important to the choreographer? Did the theme express something to which many people can relate? Why or why not?

3. What ideas were expressed in the dance for you? Did the title provide any insight into the choreography? How did your analysis of the dance and the title of the work agree or disagree?

4. Was there a sense of a beginning thematic idea being established, a de-velopment of this theme, and an end or resolution that brought the piece to a satisfactory conclusion, expressing the choreographer's point of view? If not, what was unclear in the beginning, middle, or end of the work, and what might have clarified the choreographer's intention?

5. How did the choreographer use time, space, dynamics, silence-sound-music, theatrical "texture," the dancers' potential, and the performance space to establish a choreographic style?

6. Was there a characteristic style in the movement? Was the style consis-tent and coherent with the theme and ideas of the work? How would you characterize the style of the movement and how it related to the theme?

7. Was the choreographer appropriately creative in the use of movement and visual images and in establishing a compelling theatrical environ-ment? Were there moments of surprise, tension, or humor, striking memorable visual images or sounds, or moments that strongly res-onated with your own feelings? What moments in the piece stood out for you? Why?

8. Did the work succeed for you or the audience? Why?

9. Did the choreographer introduce a concept of performance that was different from what you had previously experienced? If so, in what way?

10. Did the work challenge you to think in terms of new concepts in the use of basic dance elements of space, time, and dynamics?

11. As the diverse world dances become more visible in our society, they can influence the work of some choreographers. Did the style of this work suggest any cross-cultural influences? If you are familiar with dances from other cultures, do they have an influence on your work? If so, how?

12. What are the ongoing challenges for artists working in the dance medium? How do your own goals relate to the works you are seeing and evaluating?

General Description

1. How many performers were in the work?

2. Were the performers only dancers, or were there musicians or other performers?

3. What was the genre or medium: modern, ballet, a world dance form, musical theater, circus, nightclub act, ritual, opera, film, video, or something else?

4. What was the function or purpose of the dance: recreational, entertainment, religious ritual, concert dance, or something else?

5. What were the costumes like, or how were the participants clothed?

6. Where did the performance take place: in a defined area, such as a stage, or an undefined area, such as the outdoors?

7. What kind of accompaniment was used: recorded music, live instrumental or vocal music, or no musical accompaniment?

8. Was the musical accompaniment metric or nonmetric, that is, measured or uneven?

9. What kind of music was used: classical, contemporary, or something else?

10. How were the dancers used—as soloist, in a duet or trio, or as an ensemble?

11. Did the dancers move as a group ensemble in patterns that were circular or linear, or patterns moving toward or away from the observers, left or right, or in diagonals?

Technical Considerations

1. Did the technical support generally enhance the performance?

2. Did the music, sound, words, or silence enhance the theme? Was the sound too large or too small for the work? Was the music chopped and rearranged in a way that distorted the composer's purpose?

3. Were the lighting design and execution suitable for the piece? Was it too dark to see the dancers? Did the lights overpower the movement?

4. Did the costumes contribute to or detract from the piece? Could a change of costume give an added dimension? Were the costumes manipulated well? Did they flatter the dancers' bodies?

5. Were the props an integral part of the work? Were they used in an imaginative manner? Did the dancers seem at ease with them?

6. Were the makeup and hair designs appropriate for the dance?

Performance Considerations

1. Were the dancers well trained for what they were asked to perform?

2. Did the dancers work well together during the performance?

3. Was the number of dancers appropriate for the piece?

4. Were the dancers involved with projecting the intention of the work rather than with their technique or their bodies?

5. Did the dancers seem to be well rehearsed?

6. Did the dancers seem secure and at ease with the movement and the piece?

Space Considerations

1. What was the performance space like? Was it a regular proscenium arch theater, a thrust stage, theater-in-the-round, a room, a studio, an outdoor platform, an outdoor environmental location, a building site, a television studio, or something else?

2. How was the performance transformed by theatrical elements such as lighting or in the case of an environmental setting, by natural or human-made elements present in the site?

3. How did the choreographer adapt the dance to the performance area to take advantage of a stage that was too large or not large enough, or to an environmental venue such as the seashore?

4. Because of the location, what was the relationship between the audience and the performers? How did that affect your perception of the dance? If you are seated in a theater, you will view the dance from only one viewpoint, whereas in the outdoors you might move around and see the dance from a number of viewpoints and angles.

5. If the dance was created or restaged for television, what movements and how much of the dancer's body were selected by the choreographer to be shown to the audience?

6. How did the potentials of the television medium differ from those of a live performance? How did the choreographer manipulate the movement images by using camera and recording techniques?

DEVELOPING YOUR CRITICAL FACULTIES

You may or may not like a performance, but you should be able to understand the choreographer's point of view and to appreciate the way the themes were created and developed. If you didn't like it, first ask yourself if you came with a preconception of what dance is supposed to be and this company didn't live up to your expectations. If you want to develop your critical abilities and sensibilities, you have to be open to new ideas and new approaches in dance. Remember that many of the dance movements of the modern-dance pioneers were thought strange and ugly by an audience unaccustomed to this new way of moving.

Many times, the old rules do not readily apply to a work you have seen. Remember, the established methods and rules of choreography and performance are merely a foundation to be built upon. New modes of expression are constantly being created and developed. Some dances are composed to be antitheatrical, and some are performed in spaces other than a traditional theater or proscenium stage. For these reasons alone, the shape and content of modern dance keep changing. You don't have to accept as "great" everything you see, but you should know why you consider something great, mediocre, or merely pleasing.

Like the muscles of your body, your critical faculties and perceptions are developed by being used regularly. Just as incorrect training makes muscles undesirably bulky, a closed mind impedes both your creativity and stops the flow of new ideas in your evaluations and in your own work.

Keep in mind that as a member of the audience you are a vital part of the process of the art. The choreographer, the performers, and you collaborate in the completion of the work. The choreographer offers a vision that is created through the dancers and is given new meaning by your method of interpreting it and relating to it in terms of your own experiences. Your sincere attempt to really see what is happening, to understand the artist's vision, and to critically analyze the work from your own experiences will strengthen your evaluative abilities. The more dance you see and the more you practice analyzing what you see, the greater appreciation you will have for the dance, both as a critic and as a participant.

GLOSSARY

dance   pg. 109

evaluation   pg. 109

form   pg. 110

performance spaces   pg. 110

style   pg. 110

Appendix I
AUTHENTIC SELF-ASSESSMENT GUIDELINES

Two assessment sources you can utilize as you develop as a dancer are those of your teacher and yourself; both are important. The teacher's assessment will often stem from instructional goals related to the curriculum, while yours will usually relate to your own personal development and your perceived strengths and weaknesses related to curriculum goals.

You should know how you are doing from your own assessment rather than always relying on your teacher to give you feedback on your progress. In order to do that, you will need to establish personal criteria and goals to evaluate your ongoing improvement. One place to start is with a determination of how you are performing compared to your potential and compared to the learning guidelines established by your teacher. You should evaluate this in terms of

- practical technique development
- creative exploration
- cognitive skills, such as informed observation whereby you discover *how* to learn by thinking about the process as it is occurring
- ability to express your ideas about the dance
- your own problem-solving methods
- your social skills and how you work with and relate to others

Portfolios are a useful way to keep track of your progress. A portfolio is a record of your work, documenting your development over a period of time. It will help you identify what you have learned, recognize that you can learn on your own, develop your confidence in your own abilities, and respond to and articulate your own thoughts in relationship to what you have learned. You might want to begin by establishing a *table of contents* for your portfolio and dividing it into specific categories. Then in separate manila folders you might include

- a collection of articles you have read or handouts from the teacher
- audiotapes
- sketches you have made, graphics, photographs, or other artwork
- journal entries and ideas you have about your feelings and dance

- dance critiques of live or video performances
- daily assignments
- vocabulary acquisition
- dance quizzes and exams, moving or written
- regular class participation, punctuality, and meeting deadlines
- choreographic or improvisational assignments and creative risk taking
- peer evaluations
- scoring or evaluative charts outlining your progress

Establish a *scoring guide* that accurately reflects and measures important and meaningful achievements related to your personal goals. Determine the ways you can positively reinforce your improvements. Be objective in your self-evaluation, recognizing that there are learning plateaus. At times there may be a rush of new ideas and achievements followed by a slow learning plateau that gives you a chance to reflect more deeply on what you have learned and where you are going.

Following are examples of scoring guides that might be models for developing your own assessment. They are intended only as guides and should be modified and used only if they fit your needs.

SAMPLE: DAILY LOG TECHNIQUE CLASS

1. What was the focus of the class?
2. What was my level of participation? Did I participate fully and cooperatively?
3. What were my successes and challenges?
4. What should I work on to improve my technique or creative skills?
5. What new vocabulary word(s) did I learn? What do they mean?
6. What have I learned in class, and what have I learned on my own?
7. Were there new and unfamiliar movement sequences?
8. When appropriate, did I take advantage of working with others by both listening to them as well as articulating my own ideas?

SAMPLE: TECHNIQUE EVALUATION

Scoring skill guide levels:

5 = far above basics, 4 = above basics, 3 = basic, 2 = below basics, 1 = far below basics

Movement vocabulary that might be used in your evaluation:

alignment	breath	jumps	plié
balance	center	movement	spatial design
barre	combination	phrase	turns
body design	dynamics	music phrase	warm-up
body lines	floor work	pathways	

Movements and how you may evaluate them during a log entry:

1. Alignment: standing, bending the knees, on the balls of the feet, jumping, turning: _____ (apply scoring skill guide level)

2. Balance: on one leg, descending to the floor or rising from the floor, turning: _____ (apply scoring skill guide level)

3. Jumps: preparation, in the air, landing: _____ (apply scoring skill guide level)

4. Turning: maintaining body posture, use of arms and head, direction of rotation on floor, standing, or in the air: _____ (apply scoring skill guide level)

5. Plié: knees over toes, maintain alignment, appropriate outward rotation of legs (not forced turn-out), head-tail-heel connection (that is, awareness of the relationship of the spine from the cervical spine to the "tail bone" to the heel): _____ (apply scoring skill guide level)

6. Breath: conscious use of the breath to support the movement, not holding the breath, breath as part of the movement phrase: _____ (apply scoring skill guide level)

7. Movement phrase: visualizing the phrase, finding the essence of the phrase, use of appropriate dynamics, correctly starting the phrase, following the arc of the phrase to a successful conclusion: _____ (apply scoring skill guide level)

8. Musical phrase: starting and stopping with the music, using the rhythmical structure to support the movement phrase, listening to the music, understanding the relationship between the music and movement: _____ (apply scoring skill guide level)

SAMPLE: SELF-ASSESSMENT GLOBAL VIEW

Movement Skills

What are my strengths as a dancer?

What needs improving?

What can I do to develop my movement skills?

What can I do to develop expressive dynamic phrasing when moving?

How can I develop my ability to observe the natural sequence and flow of a phrase as well as its nuances?

Cognitive Skills

How can I become a better listener to what is being said or asked for in class or in assignments?

How can I become more of a participant in classroom discussions? Do I express my ideas about movement, do I carefully observe movement, and can I conceptualize movement and make connections to other art forms or other life situations?

Am I totally applying my thinking skills to solving the demands of the technique or creative class and using these skills to creatively problem solve in other areas of my studies or daily life?

Creative Process/Skills

Am I willing to take creative risks in choreographing, improvising, or performing, without concern about how others are going to react to my creative choices?

Am I learning the skills and choreographic methods that can make me a better choreographer?

Am I being sensitive to others and my own inner voice in improvisational assignments?

Am I sharing my ideas and listening to others regarding their ideas related to the creative process and what is being shown as a project?

Am I using the creative skills learned in dance to problem solve in other areas of my life?

Social Relationships/Skills

Am I giving my best to make the classroom experience meaningful, not only for me but also for the teacher and fellow students?

Am I working cooperatively with my peers, listening to their ideas, and sharing my own?

Am I fully engaged in the learning experience?

Do I make connections to dance as a cultural and historical event that links people of diverse backgrounds across geographical and political boundaries?

Am I learning to critically look at dance works from many perspectives: cultural, movement vocabulary, genre, dancers, choreographer, stage elements — from lighting to sets and costumes?

Some general thoughts and guidelines for the portfolio:

- Be encouraging to yourself. Assessments measure and test your personal growth. Don't be hard on yourself; the portfolio is a tool to learn about your own individual learning style and time frame. Don't compare yourself to others. Each person is unique and learns and develops in his or her own way.

- Be supportive of yourself and other students. When you work with your peers, you help one another to positively reinforce each other's learning skills and progress.

- Be clear on your personal goals and what you want to achieve — that is the value of journal writing. Identify the nature of the tasks assigned to you and what you need to do to accomplish those tasks.

- Be flexible. Not all students have to proceed through the assessment at the same rate and in the same manner. Keep your focus on the fact that you will proceed at your own pace.

- Be reflective. Whenever possible engage in positive self-evaluation and redefine your goals when you have achieved earlier goals.

- Be fair to yourself. Give yourself time to meet your goals. Keep reminding yourself that it is a process and that you can eventually meet your goals if you keep doing your best work at all times.

Appendix II
WEBSITE REFERENCES

ANATOMY/KINESIOLOGY/SOMATIC

www.Anatomyinclay.com

www.bio.psu.edu/faculty/strauss/anatomy/skel/skeletal.htm

www.Brockport.edu/~dance/somatics

www.gwc.maricopa.edu/class/bio201/muscle/mustut.htm

www.iadms.org

DANCE ORGANIZATIONS/MISCELLANEOUS

www.benesh.org/frames.html

www.Contactquarterly.com

www.cyberdance.org

www.Dancemagazine.com

www.Dancenotation.org

www.musiccenter.org/education/

DANCE RESOURCES

www.dancer.com/dance-links/modern.htm

dir.yahoo.com/arts/performing_arts/dance/modern/
    modern_companies/

www.hawaii.edu/emailref/internet_resources/Dance.htm

www.sapphireswan.com/dance/links/modern.htm

DANCE WEAR

www.allaboutdance.com

www.Capeziodance.com

www.Dancedistributors.com

www.Danskin.com

www.Leosdancewear.com

www.Nydancewear.com

FLOORS/BARRES/MIRRORS

www.Danceequipment.com

www.En-pointe.com

www.Harlequinfloors.com

www.Stagestep.com

HISTORY

www.artslynx.org/dance/history.htm

www.danceheritage.org

www.dance.ohio-state.edu/Dance_History

www.people.cornell.edu/pages/jgv4/dance/fore.htm

www.pitt.edu/~gillis/dance/disp.html

www.SDHS.org

MUSIC

www.Asgardprod.com

www.Balletclassmusic.com

www.Cathyroe.com

www.Danceclassmusic.com

www.Finisjhung.com

highered.mcgraw-hill.com/sites/0072287683/

VIDEO/DVD/CATALOGS/BOOKS

www.Dancehorizons.com

www.Facets.org

www.Kultur.com

www.Nycballet.com

www.Stottpilates.com

www.Teachersvideo.com

www.Urbankind.com

Selected References

PREPARATION

Ambrosio, Nora. (1994) *Learning about Dance: An Introduction to Dance as an Art Form and Entertainment.* Dubuque, Ia.: Kendall/Hunt Publishing Company.

Buckroyd, Julia. (2000). *The Student Dancer.* London: Dance Books.

Cheney, Gay. (1989). *Basic Concepts in Modern Dance: A Creative Approach.* Princeton, N.J.: Princeton Book Company.

DeMille, Agnes. (1962). *To a Young Dancer.* Boston and Toronto: Little, Brown.

Hannaford, Carla. (1995). *Smart Moves: Why Learning Is Not All in Your Head.* Arlington, Va.: Great Ocean Publishers.

Minton, Sandra Cerny. (1989). *Body and Self, Partners in Movement.* Champaign, Ill.: Human Kinetics Books.

ANATOMY

Berardi, Gigi. (1991). *Finding Balance: Fitness and Training for a Lifetime.* Princeton, N.J.: Princeton Book Company.

Calais-Germain, Blandine. (1993). *Anatomy of Movement.* Seattle: Eastland Press.

Caldwell, Chris. (2001). *Dance and Dancer's Injuries.* Chichester, England: Corpus Publishing.

Chmelar, Robin D., and Sally S. Fitt. (1990). *Diet: A Complete Guide to Nutrition and Weight Control.* Princeton, N.J.: Princeton Book Company.

Clarkson, Priscilla M., and Margaret Skrinar. (1988). *Science of Dance Training.* Champaign, Ill.: Human Kinetics Books.

Fitt, Sally Sevey. (1996). *Dance Kinesiology.* New York: Schirmer Books, Division of Macmillan.

Howse, Justin, and Shirley Hancock. (1992). *Dance Technique and Injury Prevention.* New York: Theatre Arts Books.

Huwyler, Josef S. (1999). *The Dancer's Body.* Germantown, Md.: International Medicine Publishing.

Iknoian, Therese. (2000). *Mind-Body Fitness for Dummies.* Foster City, Calif.: IDG Books Worldwide.

Laws, Kenneth. (2002). *Physics and the Art of Dance: Understanding Movement.* New York: Oxford University Press.

Ryan, Allan J., and Robert E. Stephens. (1988). *The Dancer's Complete Guide to Healthcare and a Long Career.* Princeton, N.J.: Princeton Book Company.

Solomon, Ruth, John Solomon, and Sandra Minton, eds. (1990). *Preventing Dance Injuries: An Interdisciplinary Approach.* Reston, Va.: American Alliance for Health, Physical Education, Recreation, and Dance.

Vincent, L. M. (1979). *The Dancer's Book of Health.* Kansas City, Mo.: Sheed Andrews and McMeel, Subsidiary of Universal Press Syndicate.

122

Vincent, L. M. (1989). *Competing with the Sylph: The Quest for the Perfect Dance Body,* 2d ed. A Dance Horizons Book. Princeton, N.J.: Princeton Book Company.

Watkins, Andrea, and Priscilla M. Clarkson. (1990). *Dancing Longer, Dancing Stronger: A Dancer's Guide to Improving Technique and Preventing Injury.* Princeton, N.J.: Princeton Book Company.

HISTORY

Anderson, Jack. (1992). *Ballet & Modern Dance: A Concise History,* 2d ed. Princeton, N.J.: Princeton Book Company.

Au, Susan. (1988). *Ballet and Modern Dance.* New York: Thames and Hudson.

Cohen, Selma Jean. (1992). *Dance as a Theatre Art: Source Readings in Dance History from 1581 to the Present.* Princeton, N.J.: Princeton Book Company.

Jowitt, Deborah. (1989). *Time and the Dancing Image.* Berkeley: University of California Press.

Kraus, Richard G., et al. (1991). *The History of Dance in Art and Education,* 3d ed. Englewood Cliffs, N.J.: Prentice Hall Publishers.

Martin, John. (1980). *The Modern Dance.* Salem, N.H.: Ayer Publishing.

Mazo, Joseph H. (1983). *Prime Movers: The Makers of Modern Dance in America.* Princeton, N.J.: Princeton Book Company.

Ruyter, Nancy Lee Chalfa. (1979). *Reformers and Visionaries: The Americanization of the Art of Dance.* New York: Dance Horizons.

Solomon, Ruth, and John Solomon. (1995). *East Meets West in Dance Voices in the Cross-Cultural Dialogue.* New York: Harwood Academic Publishers.

CHOREOGRAPHY AND IMPROVISATION

Blom, Lynne Anne, and L. Tarin Chaplin. (1988). *The Moment of Movement.* Pittsburgh: University of Pittsburgh Press.

Gilbert, Anne Green. (2000). *Teaching the Three Rs through Movement Experiences.* Seattle: University of Washington.

Hawkins, Alma M. (1991). *Moving from Within: A New Method for Dance Making.* Chicago: A Capella Books.

Minton, Sandra Cerny. (1986). *Choreography: A Basic Approach Using Improvisation.* Champaign, Ill.: Human Kinetics Publishers.

Morgenroth, Joyce. (1987). *Dance Improvisations.* Pittsburgh: University of Pittsburgh Press.

Schneer, Georgette. (1994). *Movement Improvisation in the Words of a Teacher and Her Students.* Champaign, Ill.: Human Kinetics Books.

Smith, Jacqueline M. (1985). *Dance Composition: A Practical Guide for Teachers.* London: A & C Black.

Spolin, Viola. (1983). *Improvisation for the Theater.* Evanston, Ill.: Northwestern University Press.

EVALUATION AND CRITICISM

Croce, Arlene. (1982). *Going to the Dance.* New York: Alfred A. Knopf.

Jowitt, Deborah. (1985). *The Dance in Mind: Profiles and Reviews, 1977–83.* Boston: David R. Godine Publishing.

Siegel, Marcia B. (1985). *The Shapes of Change: Images of American Dance.* Berkeley: University of California Press.

Terry, Walter. (1982). *How to Look at Dance.* New York: William Morrow & Company.

MISCELLANEOUS

Brown, Ann Kipling, and Monica Parker. (1984). *Dance Notation for Beginners.* London: Dance Books.

Chujoy, Anatole, and P. W. Manchester, eds. (1967). *The Dance Encyclopedia.* New York: Simon & Schuster.

Dell, Cecily. (1967). *A Primer for Movement Description.* New York: Dance Notation Bureau, Center for Movement Research and Analysis.

DuPont, Betty, and Joan Schlaich, eds. (1977). *Dance: The Art of Production.* St. Louis: Mosby.

Hamilton, Linda. (1998). *Advice for Dancers: Emotional Counsel and Practical Strategies.* San Francisco: Jossey-Bass Publishers.

Horosko, Marian, and Judith R. F. Kupersmith. (1987). *The Dancer's Survival Manual.* New York: Harper & Row.

Jacobs, Ellen. (1981). *Dancing: A Guide for the Dancer You Can Be.* New York: A Danceways Book.

Nielsen, Eric Brandt. (1984). *Dance Auditions.* Princeton, N.J.: Princeton Book Company.

VIDEO AND FILM

Dance Film and Video Guide
Compiled and edited by Deirdre Towers (*Footnotes* 1997, Issue No. 32)
Available from:
Performing Arts Buyers Guide
2000 Hamilton St., Suite C200
Philadelphia, PA 19105
Modern Dance and Ballet on Film and Video: A Catalog
Available from:
Dance Film Association, Inc.
1133 Broadway, Rm. 507
New York, NY 10010
Phone: (212) 727-0764
Teaching Dance Improvisation
Ririe-Woodbury Dance Company
Capitol Theatre
50 W. 200 S.
Salt Lake City, UT 84101
Phone: (801) 323-6801

PERIODICALS

Ballett International (focuses on European dance)
P.O. Box 27 04 43
Richard-Wagner-Str. 33
D-5000 Köln 1

Dance Magazine (published monthly)
    10 Columbus Circle
    New York, NY 10019
Dance Magazine: College Guide
    10 Columbus Circle
    New York, NY 10019
Dance Research Journal (published biannually)
    CORD, Dance Dept., Educ. 684D
    New York University
    35 W. 4th St.
    New York, NY 10003
Dance Teacher Now (nine publications yearly)
    P.O. Box 1074
    Davis, CA 95617

Glossary

abstraction: A removal from concrete reality in which designed forms may be definite or amorphous.

acute soreness: A short-lived muscle pain occurring after a vigorous workout.

alignment: To bring body parts into proper coordination; the placement of the body so that all segments lie on top of each other to help the body move more efficiently.

anatomically: Related to body structure.

anorexia nervosa: A serious disorder in eating behavior characterized especially by a pathological fear of weight gain, leading to faulty eating patterns, leading to self-induced starvation.

arabesque: Originally a ballet term signifying a pose in which one leg is extended straight in back; when the leg is bent, it becomes an attitude.

asymmetrical: Unequal balance, as in a spiraled seashell.

audience's focus: What the dance designer wants the audience primarily to see or experience.

axis: A real or imaginary straight line through and perpendicular to a plane of motion. Moving through a plane revolves around an axis. In dance, it is the vertical (up-down), sagittal (forward-backward), and horizontal (side-to-side). Colloquially referred to as table plane turning around the vertical axis, as in a pirouette, somersaulting in the wheel plane, and cartwheeling in the horizontal plane.

barres: Horizontal handrails held while doing exercises.

basic focus: The primary objective of the work and how each part relates to the whole.

bend: To turn or be turned from a straight line or some position. In dance, to be folded as in a hinge joint (lower arm meeting the upper arm); to curl (straight fingers curling toward the palm).

body aware: Sense of the body internally and externally; the kinesthetic sense of posture, body relationships, and movement sensation in space and time with force.

127

body half: A body half action takes place when one side of the body is stabilized in order to move or mobilize the other body half. An example is a
turn, pirouette on one leg, or another example is when you hold onto a
dance barre with one hand stabilizing the body in order to use the opposite arm and leg.

breath rhythm: Appropriate breath as a support to movement.

bulimia: A serious disorder in eating behavior characterized by binge
overeating, usually followed by self-induced vomiting or laxative abuse,
or use of diuretics, or fasting.

chaîné: A 360-degree turn, changing weight on the feet during the
movement.

codified conventions: In ballet, systematically arranged positions, movements, and performance style based on the principles of the classic ideal
of clarity, balance, and proportion.

Contact Improvisation: A dance form that gained popularity in the
mid-1970s based in part on touch and the mutual exchange of body
weight, sensitivity to the demands and responses of working with a
partner to find harmonious balance, working with gravity, and implied
social context.

contraction-release: Based on exhalation and inhalation; the act of flexing
the abdominal muscles so that the center body is in a curve and the
shoulders remain over the hips (Graham).

cool-down: Slow movement to bring the body temperature down and
center the mind after a dance class, rehearsal, or performance.

core-distal: A movement that originates from the internal muscular center
outward to the extremities or from the extremities to the center. The
"butterfly" in swimming is an example of a core-distal action.

cramp: Overfatigue of a muscle; can occur from many causes.

creative process: Method or strategies employed to fully utilize the
imagination.

critical artistic eye: Ability to discern and address the important elements
in an art form.

critique: A critical analysis or evaluation of a subject, including a dance
or art work.

cumulative rhythm: Rhythmical form in which each succeeding measure
has one more beat added to it.

dance: Considered to be the oldest art form, using time, space, dynamics,
and the human body.

delayed soreness: Intense muscle soreness that occurs within one or two days after exercise; can become more severe before healing.

demi-plié: A small bend of the leg(s) while supported on one or both feet.

die and arise: Based on the counterbalance between death and life (Wigman).

double time: Doubling the basic beat.

dynamic rhythm: Qualitative changes of movement.

dynamics: The qualitative aspects of movement energy.

eurythmics: The art of harmonious bodily movement, especially in response to music.

evaluation: A judgment or determination of the quality of something, including a work of art.

expressionism: A subjective reaction of the artist's personal feeling to events or objects through distortion, abstraction, or symbolism.

extending: A return from flexion.

external focus: The appropriate expressive elements related to the theme to be conveyed.

fall-recovery: Based on falling away from and returning to equilibrium (Humphrey).

flexing: Selective movement of a body part forward or backward.

flow: To move as a liquid does, as flowing river water. In dance, movement may flow unimpeded or meet imposed restrictions of bound flow, as river water suddenly restricted by a dam.

form: The complete shape or map of the work.

gallop: Succession of leaping strides with both feet off the ground at one time.

gestures: Movements confined to a small part of the body, such as a shrug of the shoulders.

glucose: Naturally occurring form of sugar, which is the main fuel for muscle activity.

grand-plié: A deep bend of the legs, usually supported on both feet, with heels raised.

head-tail: A head-tail is maintaining the integrity of the relationship between the top of the head (particularly the atlas vertebrae) and the tail-bone (coccyx) no matter what action is taking place in the body. Hanging down from a gymnastics bar by either your hands or from your feet puts the body in a head-tail relationship. This kind of relationship needs to be maintained whether the body is longitudinally aligned (the line of the body) or off the center line.

hemiola: A regular displacement of the usual musical accent.

hop: Leap on one foot.

improvisation: Movement performed spontaneously.

internal focus: The motivation and feeling that drives the expression of the theme.

joint: Part of the body that allows the bones of the skeleton to move in various ways, for example, the elbow joint consists of the articulation of the lower end of the humerus with the upper ends of the ulna and radius (lower and upper arm). Together they make a hinge joint whose only motion is flexion and extension (bending and straightening).

jump: A jump is any kind of spring from the floor that takes you into the air. Whether you leave the floor from two feet or one foot, or land from the jump on two feet or one it changes the nature of the jump.

kinesthetic sense: Sensation of positions, movements, and tensions of parts of the body.

Labanotation: A method of recording bodily movement in dance on a staff by means of symbols that can be coordinated with musical accompaniment.

leading-following: An exercise to develop sensitivity to working with a partner in which one leads and the other follows, often facing one another as in a mirror image.

leap: To move oneself from the ground suddenly by springing or, in dance, an aerial transition from one foot to the other foot.

leotard (unitard): Tightly fitting garment that usually covers only the torso.

lighting Manipulation of existing or artificial lights for theatrical or expressive effect.

locomotor movement: A dance concept in which the dancer moves through space from one location to another.

massage: Deep tissue rubbing to loosen muscles and bring healing to involved areas of the body.

mixed meter: Musical measures (bars) with varying numbers of beats in each measure.

mobilize: A dance concept in which the body or a body part is activated. Ideally, mobilization takes place after a preparatory "recuperation" from other movements.

modern dance: An historical and traditional mode of movement based on expressive individualized, organic, original, and ever-changing artistic standards.

motif: The gist of a movement idea.

movement recall: Ability to tap into the body memory for how a movement or series of patterns felt.

movement rhythm: Rhythmical flow of personal or organized movement.

movement vocabulary: Total resources or movement experiences available to selectively create specific coherent movement sequences.

muscles: Tissue composed of elongated cells that produces movement of the body.

nonlocomotor movement: A dance concept in which the dancer moves in a fixed area of the space.

nonstructured improvisation: Spontaneous movement without a planned movement structure.

partner awareness: Sensitivity to the pattern of movement of others, or highly acute awareness to where others are in a space or moving in a space relative to where you are.

performance space: Any place that a performer, performers, choreographers, or presenters arrange to display performance works. This could be a mime displaying on a street corner or a group of dancers on an MTV set or in a monumental theater.

phrase of movement: A series of movements making a cohesive statement.

physiologically: Related to functions and processes of an organism.

pirouette: Originally a ballet term—a turn supported on one foot *en dehors* (turn in the direction of the free leg) and *en dedans* (turn in the direction of the supporting leg). A pirouette in the air is called *tour en l'air*.

plié: Bending the knees. *See* demi-plié, grand-plié.

postures: Movements involving the entire body, such as reaction to an extremely loud noise.

relevé: Springing to the ball of the foot or tip of the toe on one or both feet.

rhythmical sense: Sensitivity to the flow of musical structure and personal movement.

RICE: Acronym for the care of skeletal injuries, which includes *rest, ice,* compression, and elevation of the affected area.

rotate: A dance concept that has multiple interpretations, from turning the whole body to turning a limb from its base to extremity (twisting).

run: A dance run may be anything from a pedestrian run staying in place or covering a great deal of distance to the point that it borders on becoming a spring from the floor. It may be stylized to establish a choreographic point of view.

shift: A movement of one body part out of alignment, or moving the whole body from one place to another.

shifted accent: Accenting a musical note other than the first beat of the measure.

shin splint: A painful condition that develops along the front of the tibia from muscle fatigue, which may lead to stress fractures of the bone.

skip: A light, quick springing alternately from one foot to the other.

slide: To move or glide smoothly from one position to another.

soft tissues: The muscles, tendons, ligaments, and bursae (a small sac between a tendon and a bone); often where acute injuries occur.

sound: Any kind of organized musical accompaniment for theatrical or expressive effect.

soussou: Springing to the balls of the feet or tips of the toes on both feet from a closed fifth position.

space: The mover's perception of the space or, more concretely, how the dancer utilizes or moves through the space as perceived by an observer or as "felt" by the mover.

spatial rhythm: Spatial patterns and spatial repetitions.

spatial tensions: Countertensions in the body or space, such as roots of a tree countering upward growth of the trunk.

spiral: Any kind of movement in the whole body or a part of the body in which a free end is twisted beyond a fixed base.

sprain: A sudden or violent twist or wrench of a joint causing the stretching or tearing of ligaments and often rupture of blood vessels with hemorrhage into the tissues; normally occurs in the ankle.

sprung dance floor: Floor structured to absorb the weight of moving dancers.

stabilized: A dance concept in which the body or one part of the body is actively "held" to cooperatively facilitate movement of another part of the body.

strain: Bodily injury from excessive tension, effort, or use; normally occurs in the quadriceps or hamstring.

structured improvisation: Planned improvisation around a theme, image, or idea.

style: A specific or characteristic manner of expression, execution, or construction in an art form or period of art.

subtractive rhythm: Rhythmical form in which each succeeding measure has one beat subtracted from it.

support: The part of the body that is bearing weight, whether on the floor, with a partner, or with nonhuman stage devices.

symmetrical: Equally balanced, as in parallel guy bars.

syncopation: Displacement of accents onto beats of the measure not usually accented.

tempo: The speed of the movement or musical accompaniment; the duration of time and meter.

theme: A unifying subject or idea.

three-dimensional: Posture or movement simultaneously using the axes of up-down, side-side, and forward-backward.

tights: Tightly fitting garment, with separate legs, for the lower half of the body.

time: A concept of quantitative or qualitative duration.

upper-lower: Upper-lower actions take place when either the upper or lower body is stabilized in order to allow the other part of the torso to mobilize. An example is sitting on a chair and twisting the upper body around your longitudinal axis or lying on the floor stabilizing the upper body with arms extended to the sides with your knees bent then allowing your pelvis to roll from one side to the other.

variation: A change or deviation in form or theme.

walk: A dance walk may be anything from a pedestrian walk across the stage to a highly stylized walk perhaps on the tips of the toes, with legs bent, or any other variation that might establish characterization, mood, or dynamic intent.

warm-up: The actions of the body to prepare for movement so that a light sweat is occurring before large movement begins.

weight: Dealing with the measured weight of an object or, in dance, the amount of force required to attain an image of ethereal lightness or of bearing the perceived oppression of forces beyond one's control.

Index